BAD
MEDICINE

LAWRENCE J.
O'BRIEN

6

BAD
MEDICINE

HOW THE AMERICAN
MEDICAL ESTABLISHMENT
IS RUINING OUR HEALTHCARE SYSTEM

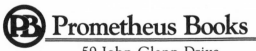 Prometheus Books

59 John Glenn Drive
Amherst, New York 14228-2197

Published 1999 by Prometheus Books

03 02 01 00 99   5 4 3 2 1

Library of Congress Cataloging-in-Publication Data

O'Brien, Lawrence J.
    Bad medicine : how the American medical establishment is ruining our healthcare
system / Lawrence J. O'Brien.
        p.   cm.
    Includes bibliographical references and index.
    ISBN 1–57392–260–9
    1. Medical care — United States. 2. Medical economics — United States.
3. Health care reform — United States. I. Title.
RA395.A3028   1999
362.1'0973—dc21   98–48718
                                                             CIP

Printed in the United States of America on acid-free paper

This volume is dedicated to Ilse O'Brien, my partner in life, and to our extraordinary offspring— William, Christina, Gretchen, and Thomas.

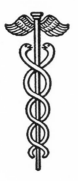

Contents

Acknowledgments   7

1. Doctors in Wonderland   9
   Pricing through the Looking Glass   12
   The Distortion of Incentives   16
   Effects of a Physician Oversupply   17
   Unlimited Expenditure   19
   Radical Reconstruction, or Collapse   21

2. A Brief Survey of the Variety of Cosmologies
   in Western History   24
   A Geocentric Universe: Aristotle,
        Ptolemy, and Dante   26
   The Almagest: Center Stage for
        Fourteen Hundred Years   28
   An Unsettler of Prevailing Dogma   32
   A Heliocentric Universe: Copernicus,
        Brahe, and Kepler   33
   Heliocentrism through the Telescope:
        Galileo   37
   A Mechanistic Universe: Descartes,
        Harvey, and Newton   40
   A Microcosmic Universe: Malpighi,
        Hooke, and Pasteur   43

An Organic, Random, Expanding Multiverse:
    Darwin and Einstein   46
A Weird New Outlook   49
The Reality of Process   50
All Science Is Cosmology   52
The Importance of Guessing Right   54

3. The American Medical Cosmos: A Clockwork Universe   58
    The Influence of a Scheme of Ideas   59
    Apprenticeship in Early American Medicine   63
    Academic Medicine in Europe   67
    The Seductive Mechanical Model   68
    Mechanism Predominates   71
    An Unbelievable Conception   76
    Persistent Resistance to Asepsis   77
    American Medicine in a Box Canyon   91
    The Important Difference Between
        Science and Technology   92
    Abraham Flexner: An Outstanding Coup   94
    Medicine's Comfort with the "Commercial Viewpoint"   102
    From the Barbershop to "Top Gun" Status   105
    Simplemindedness in the Media   110
    Radical Variation in Medical Practice   112
    A Ray of Hope Amid Intimations of Disaster   118
    A Fatally Flawed Scheme   125
    Capability and Willingness?   131

4. Legislative Remedies Increase the Illness   139
    Fee-Based Medicine:
        Serving Society's Highest Purposes?   143
    The Sky Is No Limit   146
    Oversupply Drives Expenditures   154
    More Does Not Mean Better   157
    Variation without Explanation   159
    A Chill Where Warmth Is Needed   169
    The Congressional Record   178

The Value in Buying Right   185
The Costs of Buying Wrong   187

5. What Should Be Done? Reconstruction as a Necessity   199
    Reorganization of Medical Education and
        Medical Practice   202
    Reversing the Medical Center   203
    The Importance of Generalism in Medicine   205
    Mismanaging Diabetes   205
    Public Health and Private Medicine   213
    Primary Care Is Primary   214
    Reorganizing Medical Information   223
    The Organization of Clinical Information   224
    Self-Help in Primary Care   225
    Changing Medicine's "Natural" Language   227
    Reorganizing Membership Plans   229
    Underuse and Overuse   232
    The True Measure of Value for Money   234
    Organizing Evaluative Clinical Science   236
    The Horror Story of "Practice-Style" Variation   239
    Reorganizing Economic Incentives   240
    Per Capita Payment: Enough Is Enough   240
    Lessons for Reshaping Federal Policy   243
    The Reorganization of Competition   245
    "Managing" the Competition   246
    The Significance of Clinical Outcome Measurement   254
    Concluding Precautionary Postscript   256
    Caveat Emptor   257

6. Prolegomenon to Any Future Health-Reform Proposals   263

Index   277

Acknowledgments

The author and publisher gratefully acknowledge permission to reprint from the following: From *The Discoverers* by Daniel J. Boorstin. Copyright © 1983 by Daniel J. Boorstin. Reprinted by permission of Random House, Inc.; From *The Biological Basis of Human Freedom* by Theodosius Dobzhansky. Copyright © 1960 by Theodosius Dobzhansky. Reprinted by permission of Sarah Coe; From A. C. Enthoven, "Consumer-Choice Health Plan—Inflation and Inequity in Health Care Today: Alternatives for Cost Control and an Analysis of Proposals for National Health Insurance," *The New England Journal of Medicine* 298 (March 23, 1978): 650–58. Copyright © 1978 Massachusetts Medical Society. All rights reserved; From I. R. McWhinney, "Family Medicine as a Science," *The Journal of Family Practice* 7, no. 1 (1978): 53–58. Reprinted by permission of Appleton & Lange, Inc.; From Ian McWhinney, "The Importance of Being Different," *The British Journal of General Practice* 46 (July 1996): 433–36. Reprinted by permission; From *The Norton History of Astronomy and Cosmology* by John North. Copyright ©1995 by John North. Reprinted by permission of W. W. Norton & Company, Inc. and HarperCollins Pub-

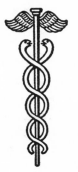

1.

Doctors in Wonderland

There is broad agreement across the land that the medical care system in the United States is in a state of crisis which, if left to fester much longer, will threaten the economic and social stability of the nation. The causes of this clear and present crisis are manifold and, in some instances, difficult to grasp. This stubborn reality has resulted in solutions being proposed, and some being undertaken, which have covered the spectrum from the ridiculous to the sublime.

The obscurity, complexity, and variety of the underlying causes of today's crisis in medical care have led healthcare planners and legislators to wander in a wonderland in which accustomed ways of analyzing a situation are out of kilter, and in which logical thinking about the issues has been undermined.

For example, consider all of the talk among members of Congress about resolving the crisis by getting the government out of the way, and allowing market forces to operate free of regulatory interference. The majority leader of the 105th Congress has been quoted as stating that: "the market is rational, the government is dumb" (http://armey. house.gov/axioms.htm). The bedrock element of a free

9

market, however, is a reliance on the certitude that the supply of goods or services will be determined by the level of demand for those outputs. In an unrestrained marketplace, it is an immutable postulate that demand regulates supply.

Consider next the contrasting and irreducible fact that the suppliers of
medical services, physicians, determine the demand for their own services.
Patients are not usually in a position to decide what medical care, or how
much care, they will consume. They must rely upon the supplier of medical
care—the physician—for these determinations. The medical profession has
made certain that no other actor in the American healthcare system has the
power to make a medical decision. The result is that, in the contemporary
American medical marketplace, supply is quite clearly regulating demand.
This indisputable fact renders the medical market irrational. The conventional wisdom of the moment may hold that the growth of HMOs and "managed-care" plans has significantly altered the fee-for-service basis of payment
for physician services. In fact, although estimates of enrollment in these
HMO-style plans run as high as 160 million individuals, fee-based payment
arrangements, usually involving discounting in some form, remain predominant. *AMNews,* published by the American Medical Association, reported
on January 20, 1997 that the share of physician revenue from all "managed-
care" contracts in 1995 represented 27.1 percent of total physician revenue,
a drop from 34 percent in the previous year. Most of these revenues were
based on contracts involving payment of discounted fees. Prepayment
arrangements for the full array of physician services, so-called capitation contracts like those between the Kaiser Health Plan and their affiliated Permanente Medical Group, remain a minor part of the overall pattern of physician
reimbursement. The campaign currently being waged nationally by the
AMA and its supporters against the administrative practices of HMOs and
"managed-care" plans should provide all of the evidence necessary to demonstrate that the predominant method of payment continues to be fee-for-service. In all fifty states, statutes and regulations firmly place the determination of what is medically necessary or appropriate for a given patient in the
hands of the physician attending the patient during a specific period of time.
Certainly, no duly licensed physician would allow a health-plan administrative person, whether a physician or not, to dictate to them as to what would
be medically necessary or appropriate for a given patient. Health-plan staff
members are explicitly prohibited by law from deciding the question of

medical necessity, unless they happen to be the attending physician for the patient in question, which would rarely if ever be the case. The decisions the plan staff do have clear responsibility to make have to do with the covered benefits of a given member, or patient, based on the terms of the contract under which they are enrolled in the plan. The AMA and its supporters are campaigning against these health-plan administrative practices, which, as every physician knows well, can legitimately only involve issues of *coverage and payment* for specified procedures or treatments. If capitation payment arrangements were predominant, the shoe might well be on the other foot: physicians could presumably be arguing with plan administrators that, in a specific case, and in spite of the terms of the applicable benefits contract, a certain high-ticket, labor-intensive procedure or course of treatment ought not be provided to the patient, despite their express preference, because of uncertainty on the attending physician's part about medical necessity or appropriateness. It should be clear that, in America, there has yet to be a large-scale movement away from fee-based payment for physician services.

The consequent hard reality that must be faced is that, in the fee-for-service setting, there is currently no effective limit on the level to which the "demand" for physician services may rise. These inverted and perverted "market forces," left unchecked in a fee-based and increasingly commercialized medical care system, can only lead to national bankruptcy.

As one illustrative example, even in such specialties as diagnostic radiology, where the referring physician would seemingly be the regulator of demand for these services, the suppliers (radiologists reading the films), through their notations and reports, have major impact on the level of demand. Current data show variations from one major metropolitan area to another as great as four times in the per capita volume and cost of diagnostic x-rays, for populations with the same demographics. These radical variations are explained only by the relative quantity of radiologists in practice within a specific marketplace, and their degree of dominance in that marketplace. A radiologist's notation: "normal, however recommend retake within thirty days to be safe," constitutes a perfect example of supply regulating demand, and presents a clear illustration of how physician income may easily be doubled by means which are virtually undetectable outside of the medical profession.

Pricing through the Looking Glass

This example also explains why a price-control strategy in medical care would be doomed to failure. In American medicine, when the unit price of a service declines in value, the units of service simply increase, so that physician income will either remain constant, or increase. There is overwhelming evidence of this phenomenon occurring continuously over the past three decades. In fact, a "top story" in the January 6, 1997 edition of *AMNews,* published by the American Medical Association, reports the following statements by Alan Hillman, MD, director of the Center for Health Policy at the University of Pennsylvania:

> Physicians aren't in the position anymore of having their remuneration go up faster than inflation simply due to competitive pressures. . . . The economic principle of "sticky down" will likely protect physician incomes from any actual declines. Things that tend not to be reduced, even under the most adverse conditions, like physician pay, are sticky down. They will never go down with respect to inflation. Managed care is going to have the leverage to command other kinds of things, like seeing more patients per hour or changing a physician venue or imposing guidelines, but physicians will draw the line at their own personal take-home pay.

Dr. Hillman was speaking about the year 1995, a year in which the same edition of *AMNews* reported a 7.2 percent increase in average physician income, over twice the rate of general inflation during that year.

Whenever physicians are confronted with the disconcerting reality of supply regulating demand in the marketplace of medical practice, and with the widespread and irrefutable patterns of unnecessary and inappropriate testing and treatment which are the consequence of a perverted supply/demand relationship, they inevitably refer to the altruistic traditions of medicine, and to the famous Hippocratic Oath which all physicians must profess upon graduation from medical school as an element of gaining the license to practice medicine.

The Greek physician Hippocrates published the first known codification of guidelines intended to govern the behavior of medical doctors. Hippocrates lived from 460 B.C.E. until 370 B.C.E. He came close to living as long as Socrates and his famous pupil Plato combined, during one of the greatest periods in Greek intellectual history. In his *Epidemics*, Hippocrates wrote:

> As to diseases, make a habit of two things: to help, or at least do no harm.

In *Dislocations*, he wrote:

> What you should put first in all the practice of our art is how to make the patient well; and if he can be made well in many ways, one should choose the least troublesome.

The Hippocratic Oath, which may or may not have been written by Hippocrates, says in part:

> The regimen I adopt shall be for the benefit of my patients according to my ability and judgment, and not for their hurt or for any wrong.

Since the publication of the Oath of Hippocrates, it is remarkable to note that there has been no other comprehensive statement produced by the medical profession, during a period of twenty-four centuries, to modify or supersede these ancient Greek guidelines.

In an essay published in 1973, entitled "The Hippocrates Myth," Martin Cherasky, M.D., delivered the following judgments on how his own profession has been doing lately in terms of its compliance with the Oath of Hippocrates:

> The myth that doctors are somehow different from other men continues to flourish . . . but we must take cognizance of the fact that money, status, and power are the forces which strongly motivate people, doctors included, in this country today. . . . Where indemnity insurance provides coverage for specified procedures, we often find the doctor's interest in his pocketbook overriding what is truly to his patient's benefit. In some localities where there is third-party payment, you can't find a tonsil left in town. Since there is no evidence that those areas have suffered widespread epidemics of rare tonsil disease, we are quite right in believing that most of these tonsillectomies should more rightly be called "remunerectomies." In the United States the surgical rate for tonsillectomies is 637 per 100,000

males. In England, where there is no financial incentive for surgery, the rate is 322.7, or just about half that number. Unnecessary surgical utilization is a tragic manifestation of poor quality care, yet study after study shows that, for all too many doctors, the temptation to equate cash with care is too strong to resist.[2]

It is nearly a quarter-century since Dr. Cherasky published those words, and things have only gotten worse since then. The silent assent of the so-called medical establishment to the virtual abandonment of the forty million Americans who today lack routine access to a physician because they do not have health insurance is all the evidence needed to support the conclusion that, in the United States today, economic self-interest motivates physicians at least as strongly as it does other people.

The population of the United States today constitutes less than 5 percent of all of the people on earth. Yet, the United States produces nearly 50 percent of the world's goods, and 85 percent of the world's energy supply. At present, our nation is spending 14 percent of its gross domestic product on medical and health care, the highest rate of expenditure by far among the nations of the industrialized world, yet forty million people are left out.

In his book entitled *Head To Head*, MIT professor of economics Lester Thurow wrote:

> [T]he United States starts the twenty-first century with more real assets that can be deployed in the twenty-first century's economic competition than anyone else. Technologically, it is seldom far behind and often still far ahead. Its per capita income and average productivity are second to none. Its college-educated work force is the best in the world; its domestic market is far larger than that of Japan and far more homogeneous than that of Europe.[3]

How is it possible that a people of such evident productive capacity and genius could have tripped so badly when it comes to the structure and functioning of such a huge and pivotal ingredient of its economic system as the provision of medical, hospital and healthcare services?

According to the 1997 report from the Office of the Actuary of the Health Care Financing Administration, the annual per capita outlay for medical care in the United States has skyrocketed by 2,000 percent over the past thirty years, from $204 per capita in 1965 to $4,100 per capita in 1995. How is it possible that, while expenditures for medical care have increased so dramatically, so many of the statistics on the health status of the population have declined so significantly?

These things have been possible because the intellectual base on which medical inquiry, medical education, and the practice of medicine have been founded in the United States has been and remains fundamentally and severely flawed. As a direct result of the erroneous *scheme of ideas* on which American physicians have relied, critical decisions which have been made regarding the selection, training, and production of physicians; the content of academic curricula; the focus and financing of medical research; the way in which the medical hierarchy has been arranged; and the professional preferences and "style" exhibited in contemporary physician practice patterns, all essentially reflect this underlying flaw.

These things have been possible because medical technology has been and is being confused with true medical science, and is in fact being marketed to the public today by the medical profession as if advances in technology define state-of-the-art medical science.

A single, recent example of what true medical science has accomplished will illustrate this point. The discovery by Barry Marshall, M.D., and his colleagues that a bacterium, *helicobacter pylori,* was the cause of stomach ulcers has eliminated all stomach ulcer surgery; all vagotomies; all psychiatric and psychological interventions for a disease which physicians believed to be psychosomatic; in fact all treatments other than a 10-to-12 day course of antibiotics costing about twenty dollars. This is true medical science. It took Dr. Marshall ten years to convince his profession that bacteria could, and did, live in the stomach lining, and he ended up swallowing a bunch of the bacteria and infecting himself as part of the proof. He began his effort to inform his medical colleagues about his discoveries of the cause and cure for most stomach ulcers in 1983, and the basic facts—the same facts—were finally accepted in 1993. During that decade, he was hooted off of a number of "scientific" platforms by the leading experts in gastrointestinal medicine. As information about Marshall's discovery was spread internationally by epidemiologists, it has become clear that the *H. pylori* hiding out in the lining of human stomachs is the most widespread chronic bacterial infection on the earth.

The technology breakthroughs currently being sold to the American public as the highest medical science in fact invariably involve the diseases which medicine does not know how to either prevent or cure. "High-tech" in medicine today is all about limiting pain and suffering, and prolonging life for patients whose diseases medicine cannot cure; and this aspect of medical care consumes the major portion of the available resources: person hours, machinery, and finances. Once the inventors of a new technological device or procedure have placed their product into the hands of the appropriate medical "specialists," the physicians who then proceed to employ the new tool or modality of diagnosis or treatment are positioned to be the principal regulators of the levels of demand for these new high-tech, and usually high-ticket, medical services.

These things have been possible because, during the past eight decades, America's physicians have spawned a medical guild designed to assure them absolute control over every aspect of their professional activities, including the nature and level of financial rewards which flow from those activities.

The Distortion of Incentives

What follows are the three outstanding features of American medicine that account for the pattern of radical increases in the level of expenditures for medical care in the United States:

- Supply shall regulate demand. No one other than a licensed physician is permitted to prescribe a treatment; order a service or device; or perform an examination or a procedure on a patient. In the event that nurse practitioners or physician assistants are involved in the care system, they are required by state statutes and regulations to practice under either direct or general supervision by a licensed physician. Decisions to prescribe procedures or a course of treatment beyond what they are personally licensed and authorized to provide must be approved by the supervising physician. The result is that physicians drive virtually all expenditures for medical care.
- Physicians shall always be in oversupply. There are at least 225,000 more physicians practicing in the United States today than would be

optimal for the nation. In its recent report, the Pew Commission on Health Professions states that there are over 600,000 active physicians, for a ratio of 240 per 100,000 people. The commission states that the consensus of experts is that the optimal ratio would be 150 physicians per 100,000 people, or a total of 375,000 active physicians. Since America's medical schools continue to graduate at least 16,000 physicians each year; and since, each year, at least 7,000 foreign-trained physicians obtain licenses to practice in the United States, the Pew Commission projects a ratio of 290 physicians per 100,000 people within seven years, nearly twice the level the Commission identifies as optimal.

• The dominant mode of payment for medical care shall be a fee for each service or procedure. Under this reimbursement system, there is no practical way for a physician to realize a profit from the prevention of illness or accident. With the sole exception of immunizations, which are usually inexpensive, the only sources of profit in medicine are disease and trauma. Stated otherwise, in fee-based medicine, there is no means by which a physician can benefit financially from health in their patients.

Effects of a Physician Oversupply

Annual gross expenditures for medical care in the United States are now in excess of $1 trillion. If there are at least 600,000 active physicians, then physicians are causing an average expenditure for medical and hospital services equivalent to $1.7 million per year per physician.

While unnecessary expenditures are being driven primarily by the need to assure the incomes of an oversupply of physicians, it must be recognized that a significant incidental result of a physician surplus on the present scale is to provide revenue for the hospitals and pharmacies with which these physicians are affiliated—revenue which is medically unjustified. Explicit collusion between physicians and the hospitals that serve as their workshops is not required here. Since 60 percent or more of every healthcare dollar is expended on the combination of inpatient and outpatient hospital services; and since physicians must prescribe all of these services; the conclusion seems

inescapable that a sizeable surplus of physicians actively engaged in gener-
ating income for themselves will simultaneously be producing significant
revenues for the hospital and for its in-house pharmacy, lab, and other diagnostic testing units. Most hospital administrators function under strong
incentives to encourage physicians to maximize their use of all hospital facilities and services unless those services are included under a "diagnostic-
related group" reimbursement, where payment is fixed, and no adjustment
to the reimbursement is possible. To the extent that the radical oversupply
of physicians that exists today results in instances of unnecessary or inappropriate inpatient or outpatient services being provided to patients, the hospital will gain revenues which are improper.

The American Medical Association's *AMNews* reported on January 20,
1997 that average or mean physician net income climbed 7.2 percent in
1995, to $195,500. The breakdown between male and female net income
was $205,800 for males and was $143,300 for females, about 69 percent of
what male physicians received. (General/family medicine showed median
incomes of $90,000 at the twenty-fifth percentile, compared with $230,000
for radiologists at the same percentile.) Adding physician overhead at 60 percent of average net income to the $195,500 figure results in an average gross
physician income of $312,800. The federal Health Care Financing Adminis-
tration issued a report in September 1998 showing that national health
expenditures in 1996 were slightly over $1 trillion. This report projects that
national health expenditures will more than double by 2006, to $2.1 trillion.
At an annual expenditure level of $1 trillion, the average gross income figure
for 1995 means that the 600,000 currently active physicians consumed
nearly $200 billion of the total health expenditures, or about 20 cents of each
dollar spent. The other 80 cents, or $800 billion, was spent on inpatient and
outpatient hospital services, prescription drugs, durable medical equipment,
long-term care, and other specialized services.

An average outlay of $1.7 million per year per active physician, times
the 225,000 active physicians exceeding the optimal ratio of physicians to
population, would add up to unnecessary and unjustifiable medical costs of
nearly $380 billion each year. It is startling to recognize excessive costs on
this scale. The fact that the annual national outlay for medical care is now
over the trillion-dollar level means that the expenditures generated by these
unnecessary physicians, and the excess cost they each represent, is on the

order of 38 percent of total annual outlays. Given the projected steady increase in the ratio of physicians to people, this figure is headed no where but up.

In the event that ways could be found to completely eliminate the current physician surplus, the national outlay for medical and health care would thereby be reduced by $380 billion annually. Assuming annual inflation of 9.5 percent, which is the Congressional Budget Office figure for medical expenditures, a reduction of $380 billion in current annual outlays would exceed $6 trillion over the next ten years. If only half of the physician excess can be eliminated, the annual expenditure would thereby be reduced by half of the $380 billion figure, and the ten-year savings would be $3 trillion. If the surplus of physicians can be reduced by just one-third, with expenditures declining by one-third of $380 billion annually, the reduction over ten years would be $2 trillion. Compare these figures to the potential savings resulting from a correction in the annual federal calculation of inflation in the overall cost-of-living, as proposed by Senator Moynihan of New York, among others: the senator is fond of pointing out that a minor change of 1.5 points would save the federal treasury $1 trillion over a twelve-year period.

Another way to look at the finding of the prestigious Pew Commission that there ought to be only 375,000 active physicians in the United States at the present population level, instead of the more than 600,000 presently working, is that the excess of active physicians existing today constitutes a surplus of 60 percent above the optimal figure identified by the commission. This surplus is now projected to continuously grow larger well into the next century.

Unlimited Expenditure

Given the foregoing unsettling realities, the truly shattering fact to be faced is that there is no possible way to predict how high the increase in expenditures on medical care might go in this nation. It should be as clear as crystal, however, that the potential is present for unnecessary, inappropriate and unjustifiable medical expenditures to rise by multiples of the foregoing estimated annual excess of $380 billion. If per capita medical expenditures are permitted to continue increasing at the same rate for the next thirty years as during the past three decades, the current average annual outlay of $4,100 per capita will increase to an unimaginable $82,000 annual cost per capita by 2025. If, on the other hand, we can figure out how to stop the increase in the physician-to-population ratio; to roll back the present oversupply of physicians; and to accomplish a reconstruction in financial incentives so that profit in the field of medical and health care will be primarily derived from the promotion and protection of health; then the per capita expenditure thirty years from now could be held in check.

It should be evident from these observations that the crisis in Medicare, for example, which got so much attention in the national political arena during 1996, is the direct result of an oversupply of physicians, deriving their income from fee-based arrangements in a structure within which the supplier of services determines the level of demand for those services. Medicare remains the most open-ended and generous federal fee-based reimbursement program in existence. An October 4, 1998 article in the *Washington Post*, entitled "Dozens of HMOs Quit Medicare, Patients Face Upheaval," reported that six million Medicare beneficiaries have chosen to enroll in an HMO, representing 15 percent of the total of nearly forty million Medicare beneficiaries in the nation.[4] The other 85 percent of beneficiaries have their Medicare-covered benefits paid for by private insurers such as Blue Cross who have contracts with Medicare to reimburse doctors and hospitals for these benefits, acting as the "fiscal intermediaries" for the federal agency. Some physicians accept whatever Medicare pays for a given service as payment in full. Others engage in a permissible level of "balance billing" of the patient. Most physicians in active practice today, except for pediatricians, derive a significant percentage of their income from their patients who are covered by fee-based Medicare. And even pediatricians treat disabled patients who have Medicare eligibility, despite their being under twenty years of age, which is the usual cutoff point between pediatric and adult medical care. Most medical offices prominently display a notice of their participation in the Medicare program. It would be an extremely rare occurrence for a physician to refuse a fee-based Medicare recipient as a patient. The reimbursement fee schedules used in the Medicare system remain attractive for most physicians, and payment is usually made promptly.

For any change in the Medicare program to have a realistic chance of ameliorating the current crisis, it must effectively come to grips with the forces that are driving the radical increase in medical expenditures, and driving the inflation of costs, chief among them an extreme oversupply of physicians who are the regulators of demand for their own services.

The excess of physicians in the United States today is a tangible, irreducible, and deplorable fact. The consequent expenditure estimates, counting the cost of services and treatments which would not occur in the absence of this excess, cannot be denied. The country will continue to ignore these stubborn realities only at its financial and social peril.

Radical Reconstruction, or Collapse

The brutal truth to be faced is that there is no reasonable alternative to a top-to-bottom reconstruction of "organized medicine" in the United States. Unless this is undertaken progressively and successfully in the near future, it is no exaggeration to state that the medical care system, which is intended to save our lives, will end up causing the economic and social demise of the unique American experiment. Some may argue that, with 160 million citizens covered under some form of HMO or "managed-care" health plan, the reconstruction being called for has already happened. This argument can be seen as fallacious in that, as has been noted in the early pages of this chapter, the dominant mode of payment even in these plans remains a fee for each service provided. It would be equally erroneous to assume that significant improvement has been made in these plans in terms of medical care management. With the exception of the Kaiser Health Plan and a handful of other group practice, prepayment HMOs, there has been little improvement made in terms of the alignment of physician and ancillary resources with the real medical-care needs of the covered population, especially in terms of the effective management of chronic diseases like diabetes; there has been no movement in the direction of aggressive effort to prevent disease or to promote optimal health in the covered population; and there have been only spotty attempts to gather and report reliable information about the outcomes of medical interventions for the covered population. In short, despite the growth of enrollment in "managed-care" plans, not much has changed in the usual and customary patterns of physician behavior.

A thousand books, or more, have been published during the past two decades citing the crisis in medicine, and proposing a variety of prescriptions for change. In terms of the impact that these works have had on the behavior of medical doctors, or on the performance of the medical care "system" in general, it seems accurate to assert that each of those books has "fallen still-born from the press." No one has paid enough attention to any of them to have made any difference. It is my contention that we will only grapple effectively with the crisis in American medicine when the leaders of contemporary medicine, and all those who influence or control the flow of dollars purchasing medical and health services, comprehend and accept the fact that the intellectual base upon which medical inquiry, medical education, and the practice of medicine rest in the United States today is flawed so fundamentally that the complete bankruptcy of the "system" is inevitable, and is not far off.

The intellectual origins of American medicine are to be found principally in Europe, at the outset in the feudal ideology and structures of the Middle Ages, supplemented at the turn of the twentieth century by the adoption of the mechanistic worldview spawned in the seventeenth century. The belated importation by the modern medical establishment of the then 300-year-old European explanation of the universe as a "clockwork" introduced fatal flaws into the bedrock of the sweeping reconstruction of medical education and medical practice in the United States which was undertaken in response to the publication of the Flexner Report in 1910. (More will be said about the importance of this report in chapter 3.) At the dawn of the twenty-first century, these fatal flaws remain fully in play, and are the root cause of the current severe "crisis" in American medicine. Coping with the challenges posed by the current medical crisis is going to require nothing less than a reconstruction in the scheme of ideas upon which "modern" American medicine presently rests and relies. The aims of this book are to expose the fundamental flaws which lie at medicine's intellectual base by examining their historical source; to suggest an alternative "worldview" from which this essential part of American culture, and of American economic life, can draw new insight and new motivation; and to propose a series of incremental steps to be taken which could provide ways and means of reorienting and reorganizing medical education and medical practice in the United States.

This book looks at the genesis and essence of the notion that the human body is a machine, a notion which continues to be the central element of the scheme of ideas that dominates the intellectual base of twentieth-century American medicine. Two pivotal questions must be answered: (1) What historical factors can explain or account for the critical situation in which the American medical care system finds itself in the final years of the twentieth-century? (2) On the basis of an appreciation of these historical factors, what can and should be done to ameliorate the current crisis?

The initial question requires a retrospective analysis of the complex of assumptions and presuppositions evident in Western intellectual history that can explain the course which the art and science of medicine has followed in the West generally, and in America in particular. Absent a retrospective critique of this kind, it is not likely that reasonable ways and means of reconstructing the *Weltanschauung* (worldview) of the American medical care system could be found, a reconstruction that must cover the complete spectrum from the criteria for selecting medical students and producing new doctors; to the setting of priorities for medical research to the thoroughgoing reorganization of medical information; to the honest solicitation of patient preference for elective medical and surgical procedures; to the systematic measurement, reporting, and evaluation of the outcomes of medical interventions across the entire range of preventive, diagnostic, and treatment activities.

This book concludes with a prolegomenon to any future proposals for reform of the American medical and healthcare system which could be deemed to be intelligent.

Notes

1. M. Mitka, "Physician Pay Back Up, But Two-Year Trend Still Shows Loss," *AMNews* (January 6, 1997): 1–3.

2. M. Cherasky, "The Hippocrates Myth," in *Hippocrates Revisited*, ed. R. J. Bulgar (New York: MEDCOM, 1973), p. 71.

3. L. Thurow, *Head to Head* (New York: Wm. Morrow & Co., 1992), p. 254.

4. D. Hilzenrath and A. Goldstein, "Dozen of HMOs Quit Medicare; Patients Face Upheaval," *Washington Post*, October 4, 1998, p. A1.

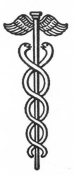

2.

A Brief Survey of the Variety of Cosmologies in Western History

A succinct survey of the cosmological theories that have influenced Western intellectual history since the time of Socrates, Plato, and Aristotle, and of the epistemological schemes resulting from those theories, is presented here as the backdrop for an analysis and critique of the erroneous medical worldview that exists in the United States today; and of the flawed medical theory of knowledge, or epistemology, which emanates from this contemporary idea of a medical "cosmos."

The word "cosmology" is derived from the Greek *kosmos,* meaning "world" or "universe" and *logos,* meaning "the study of," or "the underlying reasons for." The philosopher Alfred North Whitehead describes cosmology as

> the effort to frame a scheme of the general character of the present stage of the universe. The cosmological scheme should present the genus, for which the special schemes of the sciences are the species. . . . The cosmology and the schemes are mutually critics of each other.[1]

The word "epistemology" is derived from the Greek *episteme,* meaning "knowledge" and *logos,* meaning "the study of, or theory of." One dictionary of philosophy describes it thus:

> Epistemology is the study of the origins, the nature, the reliability or veracity and the extent of knowledge. It raises such questions as: What is knowledge? Is sense experience necessary for all types of knowledge? Is there knowledge derived only from reason? What are the differences among concepts such as belief, knowledge, opinion, fact, reality, error, imagining, conceptualizing, idea, truth, possibility, certainty?[2]

The evolution of major cosmological schemes, and of the theories of knowledge that followed from them, began with Aristotle (384–322 B.C.E.), Ptolemy (98–168), and Dante (1265–1321) as prophets of the geocentric universe; and continued with Copernicus (1473–1543), Brahe (1546–1601), and Kepler (1571–1630) as the revolutionary fathers of the heliocentric universe; with Galileo (1564–1642) as the genius of heliocentrism seen via the telescope; with Descartes (1596–1650), Harvey (1516–1650), and Newton (1642–1727) as the ingenious proponents of a mechanistic, or clockwork, universe; with Malpighi (1628–1694) and Pasteur (1822–1895) as the discoverers of the microcosmos; and with Darwin (1809–1892) and Einstein (1870–1955) as the founders of the organic, random, expanding multiverse. Each successive alteration in cosmological perspective in the West has introduced consequent alterations in epistemology which would qualify as being at least as radical as the changes in the perception of the nature and structure of the entire universe. Accordingly, this survey takes note of the variations in theories of knowledge imbedded in Western cosmologies.

My reason for asking the reader to grapple with a review of the various philosophical underpinnings of Western thought is that, in my judgment, it can provide the means to discern the sources of the present crises in American healthcare, and the means to figure out what changes in medicine's guiding "scheme of ideas" will need to be made in order to straighten out a badly disordered system, the largest and most expensive system of social services in the culture, and the system on which every citizen will eventually come to depend. Many well-intentioned attempts have been made to fix the things that are wrong with American medicine, yet there is clear and convincing evidence that the net result has been a situation that continues to worsen. The pattern of radical escalation in expenditures, which has been dampened for several years, is now displaying another pronounced burst. Serious concerns continue to be raised about the outcomes of medical interventions in terms of optimal health for patients, especially those with a chronic disease; and in terms of the quality of life, of longevity, and of medical care at the end of life. Most of the attempts at remedy during the past five decades have in fact served to increase the prevailing problems, or to create new ones. How can society, the medical profession, or those who legislate and regulate in the field of medical care possibly find a way out of this persistent mess? It is my contention that a way out of the present dilemma is to be found in a recognition of the origins of the ideas that have been driving American medicine along its present path. This recognition of origins can produce insight into how the "scheme of ideas" dominating medical thinking today has evolved into its present state of aberration and wrongheadedness. This insight into the history of the prevalent medical "scheme of ideas" can lead to an understanding of how the philosophical underpinnings of American medical practice must change, and change radically, if the immediate and pressing problems of healthcare which confront society today are to be set right within a foreseeable future. There will be a direct proportion between the degree to which the flawed content of the prevailing mind-set of American physicians can be grasped with clarity, and the extent to which real and fruitful reform of the current healthcare system can be accomplished.

A Geocentric Universe: Aristotle, Ptolemy, and Dante

Greek intellectual history presents a compelling pattern of beginning with assumptions about the cosmos, about the "ultimate stuff" or the "absolute essence" of things, and of proceeding from these assumptions to a structuring of the order of things in Nature; and then on to the elaboration of a system of logic designed to order human thinking, writing, and speaking about observations and experiences of this world.

In his *Politics,* Aristotle states: "When one says 'the Great Hippocrates,' one means not the man, but the physician." In his treatise *Ancient Medicine,*

Hippocrates wrote: "I hold that clear knowledge about nature can be obtained from medicine and from no other source." To quote Dickinson W. Richards, M.D.: "In all cases, the basis of medical care [for Hippocrates] is to understand 'physis,' that is, nature or the natural order. *The function of medicine and the physician is to assist nature to restore the balance of forces in the body, which is the state of health.* . . . Hippocrates is perfectly willing to describe a treatment that he has tried and that has failed. 'I write this on purpose,' he states, 'for these things also give instruction, which after trial show themselves failures, and show why they failed.' Where else, in ancient times, can one find a natural philosopher as disarmingly honest as this? This is not so much humility as it is respect, respect for man's fallibility, represented here in the physician, recognition that man cannot know all, that the best of his endeavors are limited, full of error."[3]

The most significant influence which the teachings of Hippocrates had upon the young Aristotle was to direct him firmly toward the intensive and extensive study of the natural order.

Historians agree that Plato's most famous student, Aristotle, was the principal architect of the foundations on which Western cosmologies and epistemologies have been erected. Consider the following brief excerpts:

> Aristotle's is . . . a mechanistic view of a Universe of spherical shells with various functions, some carrying planets. Motions were no longer being postulated as though they were mere items in a geometry book, nor were they justified in terms of Platonic intelligences, but rather in terms of a physics of motion, a physics of cause and effect. The first sphere of all, the first heaven, shows perpetual circular movement, which it transmits to all lower spheres; but what moves the first heaven? What moves it must be unmoved and eternal.[4]

> . . . [I]n the Aristotelian physics that were current until the seventeenth century it was impossible to imagine anything that could move the heavy and solid earth. And it was this difficulty in the ancient physics that caused the greatest obstruction to the scientists of the sixteenth and seventeenth centuries.[5]

Reasoning from his solid convictions about the nature and structure of the universe, Aristotle formulated the *Categoriae*, a definition of ten "categories" that formed the basis of the Aristotelian epistemology, as the foundations of a theory of knowledge that has persisted in Western thought for over two thousand years. In many ways, contemporary language and logic exhibit a heavy indebtedness to Aristotle's *Categoriae,* and to the theory of knowledge which issued from them.

The Aristotelean *Categoriae* that have functioned as the underpinning of Western language and thought for twenty-four centuries are rooted in Aristotle's cosmology, which we now understand to have been entirely erroneous. According to Aristotle, the universe was made up of four elements: earth, water, fire, and air. Earth and water moved downward, while fire and air moved upward. Being the heaviest element, earth tended to fall to the center of the universe, therefore the universe is by definition geocentric. The planets and stars, bodies above the earth and moving around the earth in perfect circles, are each imbedded in a crystalline sphere, invisible to the human eye, but accounting for the orbiting of these bodies around the earth. These crystalline spheres are moving within a fifth, often overlooked element—ether. In Aristotle's cosmology, there is no concept of empty space, and it is the ether, weightless and transparent, which occupies all that is not otherwise taken up by Sun, Moon, Earth, other planets, or stars.

At the highest level of the universe, Aristotle postulated the existence of an Unmoved Mover, or First Cause, above the outermost crystalline sphere, perfect and unchanging in its immobility, being nonetheless the principle of explanation for all motion within the universe beneath. Motion requires a mover. A cart requires a horse to pull it, or a person to push it. But all motion implies change, and the perfect cannot admit the possibility of change. From a perfect state of being, the question would be: change to what? The Aristotelean principle was that perfection required a state of rest, and that all motion implied imperfection. It is somewhat remarkable that, because of his cosmological presuppositions, Aristotle—who has been called the father of biological science—found no quarter in his theory of knowledge for the idea of process.

The Almagest: Center Stage for Fourteen Hundred Years

About four hundred years after the death of Aristotle, another great genius, Ptolemy, was born in Alexandria during the reign of the Roman Emperor

Trajan. Ptolemy's massive treatise, the *Almagest,* was clearly based on Aristotle's theories about the nature of the physical universe, and about the structure of our knowledge of the universe. It was written while Ptolemy was living and working in Alexandria, during the period in which Hadrian (117–138), Antoninus Pius (138–161), and Marcus Aurelius (161–180) ruled the Roman Empire. John North is professor of the history of the exact sciences at the University of Groningen in the Netherlands, and the author of *The Norton History of Astronomy and Cosmology.* He offers the following observations on the impact of Ptolemy's views:

> His Planetary Hypotheses went far to providing a more sophisticated version of Aristotelian cosmology. . . . The [Ptolemaic] scheme . . . became a standard part of the curriculum in Western universities in the Middle Ages. It helped inspire some of the details in Dante's *Divine Comedy.*[6]

At the time, common sense gave few reasons to question Ptolemaic theory, which may explain the endurance of his worldview, without serious challenge, for over fourteen centuries. Historian Daniel Boorstin offers this observation:

> The most influential of all ancient Roman scientists (also) proved to be the most durable authority on astrology. Ptolemy Claudius Ptolemaeus (of Alexandria) provided the solid treatise which would give substance and respectability to this science for the next thousand years.[7]

John North explains what powerful roles Hippocrates and Ptolemy played in medical circles:

> The Hippocratic writings in medicine . . . leave many hints of astrological medicine (iatromathematica), where the human body is placed under the influence and protection of the different parts of the zodiac, and of the planets. Here the logic of the argument . . . usually rested on analogies. Ptolemy describes Saturn as having a cooling and drying quality because he is furthest from the warmth of the Sun and the moisture exhaled from the Earth.[8]

The work of Dante, most notably his *Divine Comedy,* presents a clear picture of the cosmological beliefs prevalent in Western thought at the beginning of the fourteenth century. The near total dependence of the then-prevailing cosmology on the ideas of Aristotle and Ptolemy is evident in the writings of Dante.

> Dante believed in the existence of only four elements, four primary substances in this part of the universe. These were earth, water, air, and fire, and out of a mixture of them the various substances seen on this globe were held to be composed. . . . In the case of some substances you could squeeze the water out of them, and the water, when it was released, would tend to look for its true home—tend to trickle down to the sea. Substances contained the element of fire imprisoned within them, and when they were burned this fire found its escape; it fluttered upwards, seeking its true sphere, seeking the place where it could be at rest. . . . The views of Dante concerning the physical universe are really the views of the ancient world, and particularly the views of Aristotle, whom he regarded as the great master of knowledge and philosophy. Indeed, the sway which . . . Newton held over the mind of scientists in modern centuries is nothing to be compared with the dominion held by Aristotle in various fields of science for two thousand years. . . . [E]xcept in very minor details, Dante's view of the universe prevailed even into the modern centuries—it is the one which existed almost to the beginning of the seventeenth century.[9]

Daniel Boorstin describes the medical consequences of this prevalent view:

> The prevailing view of disease in medieval Europe was inherited from classical authors, elaborated by the Doctors of Physick. Disease, they said, was the upset of the balance of "humors" in the body. Medical theory was only part of their general theory of human nature. Within each person there were four "cardinal humors" ("humor" from Latin *umor*, meaning fluid or moisture)—blood, phlegm, choler, and melancholy (or black choler). Health consisted of the proper balance of these four humors, and disease came from an excess or an insufficiency of one or another of them. Each person's "temperament" was his unique balance of the four cardinal humors, hence some people were "sanguine," others "phlegmatic," "choleric," or "melancholic." . . . Since disease was a disordering of all the elements in the body, then the cures for diseases would have to treat the body as a whole. The humoral lore taught physicians how to discover the unique "natural" balance of humors in each person, and then how to restore that balance in the whole body by such treatments as sweating, purging, bloodletting or inducing vomiting.[10]

The widespread bloodletting practices of early surgeons were rooted in the astrological belief that, if a sanguine individual became ill, the way to restore him to health would be to reduce the quantity of blood in his body to the "right" quantity, so as to achieve a balance between and among the four humors. The link between cosmology and medical epistemology could find no better illustration than this. There are many other examples of cosmological beliefs dictating the content of a physicians "knowledge," and the nature of "medical" practice. In his contribution to the *Norton History of Science* series, John North made the following observations:

> The framework of formal medieval western education was based on the seven liberal arts. They provided the staple curriculum of the universities, and were a great source of strength for that characteristically European institution. . . . The faculty of "Arts" was basic, while the higher university faculties of Law and Medicine . . . were reached by a very small fraction of the university population. The vast majority of students were obliged to know the "four sciences," of which astronomy was one. Medicine in any case required a knowledge of astronomy, for not only were such practices as blood-letting related to the phases of the Moon, but astrological prognostication was an important part of the physician's repertoire. . . . One especially interesting manuscript . . . contains a collection of five horoscopes, very carefully drafted (. . . for Charles V of France), one for Charles himself and the others for four of his children. Such natal horoscopes could be consulted by the physician-astrologer at later stages in a person's life to pronounce on the probable cause of an illness. . . . [A]strologers were often primarily medical men, and when they were not, it has to be said that their salaries were much lower than those of their medical colleagues.[11]

The horoscopes were drafted for the French king by an influential bishop named Nicole d'Oresme (1330–1382) who loved to dabble in the scientific discourse of his day. Bishop d'Oresme is credited with coining the famous metaphor, "A clockwork universe, God the perfect clockmaker! . . . [I]f anyone should make a mechanical clock, would he make all the wheels move as harmoniously as possible?"[12] By the end of d'Oresme's life, a little over two dozen universities were in competition for the best and brightest minds of Europe, none of them very large, and many of them in the early stages of developing their faculties. North commented as follows about the geographic distribution of universities during this active period in European academic evolution: "Apart from Prague and Vienna, there was nothing that was both east of Paris and north of the Alps. By 1500, there are nearly fifty more foundations to be added to the list."[13]

An Unsettler of Prevailing Dogma

During the early sixteenth century, the trailblazer in medicine was a man named Theophrastus Philippus Aureolus Bombastus von Hohenheim (1493–1541), a Doctor of Physick who called himself, and who became widely recognized as, Paracelsus. His life can be seen as a continuous straying from the beaten path. He studied, but did not pursue a university degree. Daniel Boorstin writes that Paracelsus learned from his physician father, and from men of the church who knew medicine and astrology; that although he evidently did not earn a degree in medicine, he had a prosperous private medical practice in his native Switzerland; and that, at the age of thirty-three, he gained appointment as a professor—a Doctor of Physick—at the university in Basel.[14] Paracelsus was adept at self-promotion, conducted in a bombastic manner. There is speculation among linguistic scholars that the adjective "bombastic" may have been derived from his name Bombastus. Boorstin made the following observations about Paracelsus:

> [H]e seized this lucky opportunity in Basel to blast the medical establishment. At the same time, he issued his own belligerent manifesto for the healing arts which he hoped would take the place of the traditional hippocratic oath. Just as Luther ten years earlier had appealed to the primitive Church, so Paracelsus appealed over the heads of the bishops and cardinals of medicine to the pristine principles of medicine. He showed that he meant business by throwing a copy of Galen's works and of Avicenna's revered *Canton* into a student bonfire on St. John's Day, June 24, 1527. And he boldly announced that his courses in medicine would be based on his own experience with patients.[15]

What led Paracelsus to the conclusion that direct experience should be elevated above tradition in the study and practice of medicine was his faith in God, and his firm belief that, since God had created the human body, it had to be infused with an orderliness the origin of which was divine. With this inspiration driving him, the youthful Paracelsus rocked the established medical belief system to its foundations, and in doing so foreshadowed the enormous changes that occurred centuries after his death, with the beginnings of what we now call "modern" medicine. Boorstin wrote of Paracelsus's impact:

> Paracelsus' original concept of disease, despite—or because of—its mystic source, would provide axioms for modern medicine. . . . The cause of disease, Paracelsus insisted, was not the maladjustment of the bodily humors within a person, but some specific cause outside the body. "Humors" and "temperaments" he ridiculed as figments of the learned imagination. . . . When God ordered the whole universe, according to Paracelsus, He provided a remedy for every disorder. The causes of disease were mainly minerals and poisons borne from the stars in the atmosphere. This insight Paracelsus cast in his own revised language of astrology. When he pointed outside the body, when he insisted on the uniformity of causes and the specificity of diseases, he was pointing the way to modern medicine. . . . Why should not doctors use *all* the resources that God had created—mineral as well as vegetable and animal, inorganic as well as organic—to cure the body's ills? . . . "Each disease has its own physic." Who dared say that minerals and metals should not heal? . . . The objection that inorganic materials were 'poison' because they were foreign to the body was quite silly, Paracelsus observed, since "every food and every drink, if taken beyond its dose, is poison."[16]

It is worthy of note that few so-called modern physicians or pharmacologists would quarrel with Paracelsus's thinking that "Each disease has its own physic"; or with his notion that *all* of the resources that God had created—mineral, vegetable, animal; inorganic as well as organic, should be used to cure the body's ills.

A Heliocentric Universe: Copernicus, Brahe, and Kepler

Working at the same time as Paracelsus was the Polish genius, Nicolaus Copernicus (1473–1543). Here was another man who, although he was perceived as shy and timid and not at all bombastic, did not fear to confront established belief and authority on the grandest of scales. The cosmological beliefs that Copernicus developed would do no less than take the Ptolemaic universe, which had prevailed without serious question for over fourteen centuries, and turn it on its head. The earth was not the center of the universe, but was a planet in orbit about the true center, the sun. His conception of things was a direct and devastating contradiction of the established dogma of the Church; it refuted what the professors were teaching in the universities of Europe; it contradicted the astronomers of his time, most of whom embraced the teachings of Ptolemy and Aristotle; and it confounded common sense, the clear evidence seen each day, that the sun rose and set while the earth seemed to stand quite still. Here may be found the reasons why Copernicus determined that his revolutionary cosmological discoveries should not be published while he lived. When his central work, *On the Revolution of the Celestial Spheres,* was published upon his death in 1543, it was immediately placed on the Index of Forbidden Books, and remained there for two hundred years. Sir Henry Dale, former director of the British National Institute for Medical Research, had these observations about the period when Copernicus died:

> Within one month in the year 1543 there had been two events of tremendous significance in the history of science. Copernicus had laid the foundation of modern astronomy with his scheme of the motions of the earth and the planets, and the Belgian known as Vesalius, who had been a Professor of Surgery in Padua, published his book on "The Structure of the Human Body," giving the first full and accurate description of its anatomy, based on actual dissections. And then Galileo, another Padua Professor, had used the method of experiment to investigate the laws of motion and had discovered the moons of Jupiter with a simple telescope; and the memory of these great men must still have been cherished in Padua when the young Harvey arrived there to complete his medical education, after he had studied at Caius College in Cambridge.[17]

In turning the cosmos upside down, Nicolaus Copernicus provided a new, deeply challenging framework for Western thought to grapple with, not merely in the fields of cosmology, astronomy, and astrology, but along the entire range of intellectual inquiry. In his work *The Copernican Revolution,* Thomas Kuhn makes cogent note of this fact:

Conceptions like [Niels] Bohr's atom and [Albert] Einstein's finite but unbounded space were introduced to solve problems in a single scientific specialty. . . . Every fundamental innovation in a scientific specialty inevitably transforms neighboring sciences and, more slowly, the worlds of the philosopher and the educated layman. Copernicus's innovation is no exception. In the early decades of the seventeenth century it was at best an astronomical innovation. Outside of astronomy it raised a host of problems just as perplexing and far more obvious than the questions of numerical detail it had resolved. Why do heavy bodies always fall toward the surface of a spinning earth as the earth moves in its orbit about the sun? How far away are the stars, and what is their role in the structure of the universe? What moves the planets, and how, in the absence of spheres, are they kept in their orbits? Copernican astronomy destroyed traditional answers to these questions, but it supplied no substitutes. A new physics and a new cosmology were required before astronomy could again participate plausibly in a unified pattern of thought.[18]

The next significant progression in the evolution of Western cosmological theory came at the hands of a Danish astronomer, Tycho Brahe (1546–1601). Boorstin has made the following observations about Brahe's education:

[B]orn just three years after Copernicus died. . . . Tycho Brahe (1546–1601) . . . was introduced to all seven of the liberal arts—the trivium (grammar, rhetoric and logic) and the quadrivium (geometry, astronomy, arithmetic, and music). . . . Of course he studied astrology, an "interdisciplinary" study combining astronomy and medicine, which made astronomers seem useful in everyday affairs.[19]

Despite his classical preparation as a professional student of mathematics, astronomy, and astrology, Brahe was an inveterate tinkerer, and was extremely good with his hands. He used such basic instruments as an ordinary compass of the sort used by a draftsman, and a "cross-staff," which consisted of two graduated rods, one twice the length of the other, with the shorter rod able to be slid up or down the longer rod, arranged so as to form a right angle between them. He used his handmade instruments to measure and to remeasure. He made and carefully kept comprehensive records of every calculation and recalculation. What his efforts told him was that there were flaws in Ptolemy's conception of the universe, on the one hand; and that, on the other hand, his own measurements could not confirm the new-fangled conception published by Copernicus. Boorstin describes Brahe's conclusions as follows:

> Tycho devised his own compromise with its own kind of simplicity. He left an unmoving earth at the center while the sun continued, as in the Ptolemaic system, to go around the earth. But in Tycho's new scheme, the other planets rotated around the Sun following the sun's movements about the earth.[20]

The Danish monarch, King Frederick II, gave Brahe a two-thousand-acre offshore island from which he could conduct his astronomical observations. He also provided a financial subsidy to support Tycho's work. According to Daniel Boorstin, Brahe made his heavenly observations

> with scrupulous regularity, repeating them, combining them, and trying always to allow for the imperfections of his instruments. As a result he reduced his margin of error to a fraction of a minute of an arc, and provided the sharpest precision achieved by anyone before the telescope.[21]

When Brahe realized that he was dying and would not have the time to flesh out his own theory of the structure of the universe, intended as the alternative to both the Ptolemaic and the Copernican theories, he invested his hopes and expectations in a man twenty-five years younger than himself, a German astronomer and mathematician named Johannes Kepler (1571–1630). Tycho Brahe gave all of his books and records to Kepler, an act which determined the direction in which all of Kepler's energies would henceforth be invested. Kepler grounded his own astronomical observations and mathematical formulations in his theological beliefs, in particular his belief that the Creator had bequeathed us a world shot through with harmonies, if we could but learn to perceive and understand them. Boorstin made these observations about Kepler's work:

> His first book, . . . the *Mysterium Cosmographicum* (1596), was a *tour de force* of mathematical mysticism, and set the course for his lifework. . . . [T]his book by the twenty-five-year-old Kepler a full half-century after Copernicus' *De Revolutionibus* was the first outspoken defense of the new system

after Copernicus himself. . . . When Kepler tried to account for the decrease in the linear velocity of a planet as its distance from the sun increased, at first he . . . imagined that each planet had its own "moving spirit." . . . Kepler . . . later momentously added that his whole system of celestial physics made perfect sense "if the word soul (anima) is replaced by force (vis)." So he boldly pointed the way from an organic to a mechanical explanation of the universe. . . . Might it not be possible, Kepler asked, "to show that the celestial machine is not so much a divine organism but rather a clockwork . . . inasmuch as all the variety of motions are carried out by means of a single very simple magnetic force of the body, just as in a clock all motions arise from a very simple weight?"[22]

As the sixteenth century came to a close, the brilliant Kepler, building on the extraordinary body of work passed on to him by Brahe, had taken cosmological inquiry just as far as the naked eye could go. He had also propagated his view of the universe as "a celestial machine," a view which would illuminate the thinking of another great mathematician, René Descartes, eventually leading to the seventeenth-century embrace of a frankly mechanistic universe, bifurcated in terms of matter and mind. Within this Enlightenment cosmology, to which Kepler contributed in significant measure, lies the root system of the flawed "scheme of ideas" that is the philosophical and intellectual base of conceptualization for the leaders of contemporary American medicine.

Heliocentrism through the Telescope: Galileo

Galileo Galilei (1564–1642) was born in the town of Pisa. He was seven years older than Johannes Kepler, and he lived eleven years after Kepler's death. Galileo began his university career in Padua, where he enrolled as a student of medicine. While teaching mathematics at the University of Padua, Galileo maintained an artisan shop in town. Like Kepler, he designed and produced various instruments for measuring and surveying. In addition to sextants and compasses, he engaged in the manufacture of telescopes as a sideline, initially for commercial purposes. He provided looking glasses to the maritime industry for use in navigation on both merchant and military sailing vessels. As his proficiency in grinding and assembling lenses improved, he eventually thought of using his new instruments to observe the heavens. Daniel Boorstin has commented about this evolution in Galileo's use of his telescopes:

> [I]f Galileo had been merely a practical man, the telescope would not have been such a troublemaker. Other nations would have shared the Venetian Senate's enthusiasm for a new device that served commerce and warfare by making distant objects seem close. For some reason, however, Galileo would not leave it at that. Early in January, 1601 he did what now seems most obvious—he turned his telescope towards the skies.[23]

During the Middle Ages, disputation had been raised to a true art form in Europe, as the scholastics debated topics such as the number of angels who could fit on the head of a pin. What is often not grasped about the nature of disputation in European universities, however, is the fact that argument based in any significant manner upon direct experience and observation was utterly disvalued and rejected. A decent example is found in the tale of a Jesuit seminarian participating in a scholastic disputation concerning the number of teeth in a horse's mouth. When the young student suggested that they get a horse and count its teeth, he was summarily ejected from the seminary—turned out into the nasty and brutish world outside the walls of the monastery. The persistent and strong opposition of the Church and the universities to the Copernican revolution in cosmology, even in the face of telescopic evidence, demonstrated that perceptions of the value of direct observation or direct experience had changed very little. As Thomas Kuhn has observed:

> Kepler's ellipses and Galileo's telescope did not immediately crush the opposition to Copernicanism. . . . [N]ot until the last decades of the seventeenth century did Kepler's Laws become the universally accepted basis for planetary computations even among the best practicing European astronomers. Galileo's observations met initially even greater opposition. . . . With the advent of the telescope Copernicanism ceased to be esoteric. The telescopic discoveries . . . provided a natural and appropriate focus for much of the continuing opposition to Copernicus' proposal. They showed the real cosmological issues at stake more quickly and more clearly than pages of mathematics. . . . The continuing opposition to the results of tele-

scopic observation is symptomatic of the deeper-seated and longer-lasting opposition to Copernicanism during the seventeenth century. Both derived from the same source, *a subconscious reluctance to assent in the destruction of a cosmology that for centuries had been the basis of everyday practical and spiritual life.*[24] (Emphasis added)

The telescope made all the difference for Galileo. He could see the arrangement of heavenly bodies for himself. However, when it came to disputation with established authority over the way things really are, direct observation of the heavens proved of no earthly use to him in conducting these arguments. Because Galileo and his telescope provided the Western world with visual evidence that the earth was not the center of the universe, he was threatened and hounded into silence. During the first quarter of the seventeenth century, Galileo was forced out of his professorship at the University of Pisa for teaching his students about the work of Copernicus. Galileo published his *Dialogue on the Two Chief World Systems* in 1632, presenting the evidence in support of a heliocentric cosmology, based upon the revolutionary discoveries flowing from his astronomical observations. The Roman Church, along with the centers of learning in Italy and other European countries, swiftly condemned Galileo's writings. The Church forbade him from teaching about his discoveries, and placed his work on the Index of Forbidden Books. During much of this period, which Alfred North Whitehead has termed the "Century of Genius," the insistent message being transmitted to innovative scientists was that, in any fundamental dispute over the order of things in the natural universe, argument based on authority would always take precedence and prevail over argument based upon demonstrable experience. During the seventeenth century, and ever since, the field of medicine seems to have consistently exhibited a strong affinity for this particular viewpoint about the proper relationship between authority and experience.

At age sixty-nine, the great genius Galileo knelt before the pope's tribunal in Rome and, perhaps with his tongue firmly planted in his cheek, retracted his own published theory of the cosmos and recanted all of the facts he had uncovered and understood via his direct experiences with the telescope.

I, Galileo, son of the late Vincenzio Galilei, Florentine, aged seventy years, arraigned personally before this tribunal and kneeling before you, Most eminent and Lord Cardinals Inquisitors-General against heretical pravity throughout the entire Christian Commonwealth, having before my eyes and touching with my hands the Holy Gospels, swear that I have always believed, do believe, and with God's help will in the future believe all that is held, preached and taught by the Holy Catholic and Apostolic Church. But, whereas, after an injunction had been lawfully intimated to me by this Holy Office to the effect that I must altogether abandon the false opinion that the sun is the center of the world and immobile, and that the earth is not the center of the world and moves, and that I must not hold, defend, or teach, in any way, verbally or in writing, the said false doctrine, and after it had been notified to me that the said doctrine was contrary to Holy Scripture, I wrote and printed a book in which I treated this new doctrine already condemned and brought forth arguments in its favor without presenting any solution for them, I have been judged to be vehemently suspected of heresy, that is, of having held and believed that the sun is the center of the world and immobile and that the earth is not the center and moves.

Therefore, desiring to remove from the minds of Your Eminences, and of all faithful Christians, this vehement suspicion rightly conceived against me, with sincere heart and unpretended faith I abjure, curse, and detest the aforesaid errors and heresies and also every other error and sect whatever, contrary to the Holy Church, and I swear that in the future I will never again say or assert verbally or in writing, anything that might cause a similar suspicion toward me, further, should I know any heretic or person suspected of heresy, I will denounce him to this Holy Office or to the Inquisitor or Ordinary of the place where I may be.[25]

A Mechanistic Universe:
Descartes, Harvey, and Newton

In 1650, eight years after the death of Galileo, two other European men of genius passed away: René Descartes and William Harvey—Descartes at age fifty-four and Harvey at age seventy-four. Harvey was only sixteen when he began six years of medical studies at Caius College, Cambridge, in 1593, three years before Descartes was born. In 1599, he went to Italy to attend the university at Padua, where Vesalius had been a renowned professor of surgery and anatomy, and where Galileo had been both a student of medicine and an esteemed professor of mathematics. After completing his studies in Padua,

Harvey returned to England, and within a short time married into a well-positioned family. His father-in-law was a practicing physician who had attended Queen Elizabeth. Harvey gained appointment to the College of Physicians and had a flourishing medical practice. His patients were chiefly aristocrats, and his network of colleagues and associates included Sir Francis Bacon. Harvey was certainly familiar with Bacon's theories of inductive reasoning, and with the book Bacon published in 1605, *The Advancement of Learning.* C. D. Broad, formerly Knightbridge Professor of Moral Philosophy at Cambridge, has provided a summary of Bacon's thinking:

> . . . Bacon was completely convinced that the ignorance of nature and the consequent lack of power over nature, which had prevailed from the earliest times up to his day, were by no means inevitable. They sprang . . . simply and solely from the use of a wrong method. . . . The fundamental defects . . . were the following. In the first place there was an almost complete divorce between theory, observation and experiment, and practical application. Plenty of experiments of a kind had been done, and a certain number of disconnected empirical rules or recipes had been discovered. . . . [E]ven when they were (done by) honest and sensible men, they did their experiments with some immediate practical end in view, such as . . . discovering a universal medicine for all diseases. They were not guided by any general theory; . . . and they worked in isolation from each other, keeping their results secret rather than pooling them. . . . Bacon rightly accused the learned men of his time of accepting on authority sweeping general principles which Aristotle . . . had reached by hasty and uncritical generalisation from a few rather superficial observations. Using these as premises, they proceeded to deduce conclusions about nature.[26]

William Harvey's writings illustrate the influence that Bacon's methodology had on his own work. Harvey published his revolutionary work on the circulation of the blood in 1628, eight years after the *Mayflower* had landed at Plymouth Rock, and four years before Galileo published his earthshaking *Dialogue.* Harvey's work, *An Anatomical Treatise on the Movement of the Heart and the Blood,* presented brand-new and intriguing scientific information about the human organism. One might expect that Harvey's work would have been received with a sense of great curiosity and even awe, but the actual reception was quite otherwise. Forty-three years passed before the prevailing medical authorities determined, in 1671, that the discoveries Harvey had made and meticulously reported would be accepted, and added to the then-current store of medical information. Sir Henry Dale believed that, in Harvey's *Treatise*: "[W]e can find the very beginning of medical science in the modern sense."[27] During this same period, the French philosopher René Descartes was working up a new cosmological scheme of his own that would further unsettle conventional cosmological wisdom, and that would play a pivotal role in the progress of scientific inquiry during the next three centuries. Descartes wrote *The World, or, Treatise on Light*, presenting and defending the new mechanistic conception of the universe which he had been developing during the early 1630s. Knowing of the troubles that Galileo was undergoing with the authorities in Rome and with the scholarly community throughout Europe, the Jesuit-trained Descartes prudently decided against publishing his *Treatise.* Although his ideas were well known to European students of mathematics, astrology, and astronomy, the *Treatise* itself did not appear in print until after his death. Certainly among the students who were aware of the theories of René Descartes prior to their appearance in print was the young Englishman Isaac Newton, who began his studies at Trinity College, Cambridge, in 1661—three years before the death of Descartes. Daniel Boorstin has taken note of this awareness:

> When Newton went to Cambridge, the physics of Aristotle, based on the distinction of qualities, was being displaced by a new "mechanical" philosophy of which Descartes was the most famous exponent. *Descartes described the physical world as consisting of invisible particles of matter in motion in the ether. Everything in nature, he said, could be explained by the mechanical interaction of these particles. According to Descartes's mechanistic view of the world, there was no difference, except in intricacy, between the operation of a human body, of a tree, or of a clock.*[28] (Emphasis added)

As Alexander Pope keenly observed: "God said: 'Let Newton be!', and there was light." John North has said that Isaac Newton's book *Mathematical Principles of Natural Philosophy* "is considered the most important work ever published in the physical science."[29] With a heavy indebtedness to the mechanical conception of nature articulated so effectively by Descartes, Newton proceeded to establish a new framework for carrying on with research in the field of astronomy—a framework which, in North's words, marked the end of one historical era and the beginning of another. . . . [I]t presented a programme for future astronomical research that in some respects still continues. Its demonstrations were not always complete—indeed, in many cases Newton had not yet developed the necessary mathematical techniques to give compelling proofs. As later astronomers were to discover to their surprise, however, he had a remarkable instinct for correct conclusions, even when he had to paper over the cracks in his arguments.[30]

A Microcosmic Universe:
Malpighi, Hooke, and Pasteur

Marcello Malpighi lived two centuries before Louis Pasteur. He was born into a family of wealth in Bologna in 1628, and he died at the age of sixty-six. He graduated from the University of Bologna in 1653, with doctoral degrees in medicine and in philosophy. He was appointed professor of theoretical medicine at the University of Pisa, where Galileo had been a student, and later held the chair in mathematics. At Pisa, he befriended Giovanni Borelli, a professor of mathematics, known as the founder of *iatrophysics,* defined as "the application of physics to medicine."[31] Malpighi encountered Harvey's work while he was a medical student at the University of Bologna. Harvey's carefully detailed descriptions and explanations of how the heart worked and the blood circulated captivated young Malpighi, and in a significant way directed his subsequent scientific pursuits. Harvey's work showed clearly that the supply of blood in the human body circulated completely through the organism continuously, numerous times each day. One thing that Harvey's anatomical treatise had not explained, however, was where this large supply of blood was being stored, since it was pumped through the heart rapidly, and since the rate at which the body produced blood was very slow. Malpighi dedicated his time and talent to finding an answer to this difficult question. Boorstin has commented on this development:

> Until that mystery, which had troubled Harvey himself, was solved, there remained room to doubt Harvey. Malpighi located the mystery in the lungs. And there he would solve the mystery by new techniques of comparative anatomy. In 1661 he announced his discoveries in two brief letters from Bologna to his old friend in Pisa, Giovanni Borelli. These were

quickly published in Bologna as a book *On the Lungs* and became a pioneer work in modern medicine.[32]

Malpighi has been referred to as the "founder of microscopic anatomy. . . . Two looks through Galileo's telescope, Malpighi exclaimed, had revealed more of the heavens than was seen in all the millennia before."[33] He would use his own primitive optical tubes to explore the microcosmos, and he anticipated results no less spectacular than Galileo's. His methodology was inductive in that he studied the facts before him, intensively and exhaustively, and from a wealth of microscopic observations he constructed his explanations and drew his conclusions, His own clearly fertile imagination, stimulated by Harvey's writings, guided his selection of the particular collection of facts to be studied at a given time. Daniel Boorstin has provided the following observations:

> Malpighi had discovered the capillaries (and)...he revealed the structure and function of the lungs, opening the way to understand the process of respiration. . . . Malpighi's strength would be tested . . . by the envy and malice of his medical colleagues. . . . The know-nothings had refused to look through Galileo's telescope or refused to believe what they saw. The "flea glass" was so handy that it was harder for them to refuse to look through it, but they, again, objected that the microscope distorted natural shapes, added colors that were not there, and was a device for counterfeiting reality. Such attacks came from the most respectable sources, and even, to Malpighi's special pain, from his own students. . . . So much for the microscope.[34]

Robert Hooke (1635–1703) was the Secretary of the Royal Society in London during the 1660s and served as Curator of Experiments for the society. Hooke knew Newton, and he spent time on experiments with gravitation and the movements of the macrocosmos with none of the success that Newton achieved. His experiments with the compound microscope, on the contrary, led him to publish his *Micrographia* in 1665. Boorstin has commented on this event:

> What Galileo . . . had done for the telescope and its heavenly vistas, Hooke's *Micrographia* now did for the microscope. . . . [W]hat he described seeing in his compound microscope awakened learned Europe to the wonderful world within. Fifty-seven amazing illustrations drawn by Hooke

himself revealed for the first time the eye of a fly, the shape of a bee's stinging organ, the anatomy of a flea and a louse, the structure of feathers, and the plantlike form of molds. . . . Just as the telescope had brought together the earth and the most distant heavenly bodies into a single scheme of thought, now microscopic vistas revealed a miniscule world surprisingly like that seen on a large scale every day.[35]

As the seventeenth century drew to a close, Europe entered an era during which the preoccupation of its intellectuals would almost of necessity be with the digestion of the explosion of insights, hypotheses, and ideas inherited from the unusual succession of men of genius who had lived and labored during the years from 1600 until 1699. The mathematician and philosopher Alfred North Whitehead has neatly summed up the seventeenth century:

A brief, and sufficiently accurate, description of the intellectual life of the European races during the succeeding two centuries and a quarter up to our own times is that they have been living upon the accumulated capital of ideas provided for them by the genius of the seventeenth century. . . . It is the one century which consistently, and throughout the whole range of human activities, provided intellectual genius adequate for the greatness of its occasions.[36]

In the Louis Clark Vanuxem Lectures delivered at Princeton University in 1929, Whitehead had this additional commentary on the fertile seventeenth century:

Kepler produced the first important utilization of conic sections, the first among hundreds, Descartes and Desargues revolutionized the methods of science, Newton wrote his *Principia,* and the modern period of civilization commenced. Apart from the capital of abstract ideas which had accumulated slowly during two thousand years, our modern life would have been impossible. There is nothing magical about mathematics as such. It is simply the greatest example of a science of abstract forms. . . . *The point is that the development of abstract theory precedes the understanding of fact.*[37] (Emphasis added)

It was not until nearly two centuries after the publication of Hooke's *Micrographia* that Western thought gained deeper insight into the microcosmic world, thanks chiefly to the work of Pasteur. One reason for this long hiatus had to do with the primitiveness of microscopes prior to the first quarter of the nineteenth century.

> The microscope is the biologist's chief tool, and the microscopes of 1800 were not much better than those of a hundred years before . . . no one made an achromatic microscope objective until 1825.[38]

Louis Pasteur was born in 1822, when Charles Darwin was just thirteen years old. Pasteur has been a pivotal figure for many reasons, one of them being that his experiments finally sounded the death knell for the theory of spontaneous generation. As Daniel Boorstin has observed:

> [I]t was not until Louis Pasteur's brilliant experiments with fermentation in the nineteenth century, and his practical application of his ideas for the preservation of milk, that the dogma (of spontaneous generation) ceased to be scientifically respectable.[39]

As a microbiologist, Pasteur's discoveries supported the theories of Darwin, and in many ways opened pathways to the "inside" universe which paralleled the openings to the macrocosmos that would soon issue from the mind of physicist Albert Einstein. Pasteur played a pivotal part in the evolution of a new cosmology that would look inward as well as to the heavens, a cosmology of organism rather than of mechanism—a cosmology flowing from a teeming microcosmos and from a seemingly infinite and expanding macrocosmos.

An Organic, Random, Expanding Multiverse: Darwin and Einstein

An invertebrate zoologist at Cambridge, Dr. C. F. A. Pantin, has signaled the centrality of Darwin's revolutionary insights in the following sentence: "The change in our ideas of how life began was the result of a scientific revolution which followed the publication of Darwin's book in 1859."[40]

In spite of the fact that the idea of evolution has been truly revolutionary for science in the twentieth century, the following verifiable observation by philosopher Daniel Dennett speaks volumes about the general receptivity within contemporary American culture to the main feature of the Darwinian revolution: "Americans are notoriously ill-informed about evolution. A recent Gallup poll (June 1993) discovered that 47 percent of adult Americans believe that *Homo sapiens* is a species created by God less than ten thousand years ago."[41]

When Copernicus pronounced in 1543 that the sun, and not the earth, was at the center of the universe, and that the earth was in an orbit, revolving around the sun, his radical notions were resisted for more than a century. It has been noted by scholars that, in our era of sophistication and learning, while more than a century has passed since Darwin presented his revolutionary ideas to the public in 1859, the theory of evolution remains a very controversial subject for many people.

> In all his brilliant musings, Darwin never hit upon the central concept without which the theory of evolution is hopeless: the concept of a gene . . . Darwin recognized the seriousness of this challenge, and neither he nor his ardent supporters succeeded in responding with a description of a convincing and well-documented mechanism of heredity that could combine traits of parents while maintaining an underlying and unchanged identity. The idea they needed was right at hand, uncovered . . . by the monk Gregor Mendel and published in a relatively obscure Austrian journal in 1865, but, in the best-savored irony in the history of science, it lay there unnoticed until its importance was appreciated (at first dimly) around 1900. Its triumphant establishment at the heart of the "Modern Synthesis" (in effect, the synthesis of Mendel and Darwin) was eventually made secure in the 1940s, thanks to the work of Theodosius Dobzhansky, Julian Huxley, Ernst Mayr, and others. It has taken another half-century to iron out most of the wrinkles of that new fabric. The fundamental core of contemporary Darwinism, the theory of DNA-based reproduction and evolution, is now beyond dispute among scientists. . . . The Darwinian Revolution is both a scientific and a philosophical revolution, and neither revolution could have occurred without the other. . . . It was the philosophical prejudices of the scientists, more than their lack of scientific evidence, that prevented them from seeing how the theory could actually work, but those philosophical prejudices that had to be overthrown were too deeply entrenched to be dislodged by mere philosophical brilliance. It took an irresistible parade of hard-won scientific facts to force thinkers to take seriously the weird new outlook that Darwin proposed.[42]

The significance of heredity for the theory of evolution—in biological and in cultural terms—has been best expressed by the geneticist Theodosius Dobzhansky:

> Evolution is change in the heredity, in the genetic endowment, of succeeding generations. Heredity is a conservative force; it tends to make the offspring like their parents and to make future generations like their ancestors. If heredity were perfect there would be no evolution. It is a remarkable combination of stability and changeability which makes heredity the vehicle of evolution. Heredity is the basis of the biological evolution of all forms of life—from viruses and bacteria to mice and men. . . . [H]eredity is the self-reproduction of the organism *using materials taken from the environment,* and self-reproduction is life. No understanding of evolution is possible except with the foundation of a knowledge of heredity.[43] (Emphasis added)

> Man may be said to have two heredities, a biological one and a cultural one. . . . It is important to realize that biological heredity and culture, the inborn and the learned behavior, are not independent or isolated entities. They are interacting processes. . . . Human evolution is a singular product of interaction between biology and culture.[44]

> The operation of heredity in bringing about the development of a living individual occurs by means of assimilation of food and of growth. A fertilized human egg . . . (diameter 0.1 of a mm; weight 0.000,000,05 of an ounce) becomes eventually an adult person who weighs, say, 160 pounds. This is approximately a fifty billion-fold increase in weight. The tremendous increase in mass occurs evidently at the expense of the food which the individual consumes and assimilates, assimilation being a process whereby the food materials derived from the environment are chemically transformed to become the constituents of the living body. Heredity furnishes the pattern of these transformations, which build a likeness of the assimilating body *out of the materials taken in from the environment.* . . . An estimate, first made by H. J. Muller, shows how incredibly small are the material carriers of heredity. . . . All the egg cells which gave rise to the present population of the earth, about two and a half billion of them, would . . . fit easily into a gallon pitcher. An equal number of spermatozoa would have a much smaller volume, less than that of a regular aspirin tablet. . . . The

aggregate volume of all the genes in all the sex cells which produced the world's population today would probably not exceed that of a vitamin capsule. This tiny mass contains, then, all the biological heredity of the living representatives of our species and the material basis of its future evolution.[45] (Emphasis added)

A change in a single gene can so alter the course of development of the organism that, instead of a normal child who easily absorbs the elements of culture, there is produced a wretched being, unable to respond to the socializing influences of his human environment.[46] (Emphasis added)

Man is neither particularly strong in body nor particularly agile in movement. If it were not for his brain he would be a rather pitiable misfit in most environments, and would probably have become extinct long before now. It is his capacity to acquire and to accumulate experience and knowledge that made him an unprecedented biological success.[47]

A Weird New Outlook

Darwin's "weird new outlook" has had a major impact beyond the field of biology—profoundly affecting contemporary theories of knowledge, as well as underlying ideas about the nature and structure of the cosmos. The idea of *process* as essential to an accurate understanding of nature began to seep into other fields of inquiry.

Daniel C. Dennett, in his book *Darwin's Dangerous Idea,* has made the following observation about the wide impact of the theory of evolution:

Darwin's idea had been born as an answer to questions in biology, but it threatened to leak out, offering answers—welcome or not—to questions in cosmology (going in one direction) and psychology (going in the other direction).[48]

In the age of Thomas Aquinas and the schoolmen, as they were rediscovering Aristotle's writings and reconstructing his ideas within a distinctly Christian set of theological beliefs about the nature of the First Cause, one of the stumbling blocks became Aristotle's notion of the Unmoved Mover. The scholastics were confronted with the task of reconciling the Aristotelean idea of a godhead at rest, and therefore perfect, with the Christian notion of a "Triune" God, whose perfection is defined by the dynamic relationship between Father and Son, related through a Spirit—Love—which performs a function so profound as to warrant personification, the "third person" in the Trinity. Three persons, one God: here the scholastics had the idea of *process* as a defining characteristic of the godhead itself; an idea that change and motion exist within the godhead, as the Son participates in human history at a specific moment in time to express the spirit and purposes of the Father. These assumptions about the nature of the First Cause among the scholastics differed radically from the Aristotelean concepts, and inevitably conditioned their perceptions of Aristotle's teachings. This Western idea of *process* at the root of understanding the world of biology and of the microcosmos clearly fed into Einstein's thinking about the nature and essence of the macro-cosmos. Physics moved rapidly into new directions under the stimulus of the notion of *process* at the very heart of things.

The Reality of Process

John North has noted in his book on astronomy and cosmology that virtu-ally every contemporary theory about the way the universe is structured "can be traced back in part to the ideas of Albert Einstein, developed in the decade ending in 1915."[49]

Daniel Boorstin has made the following observations about the origins of Einstein's insights:

> The dissolution of the indestructible solid atom would come from two sources . . . from the study of light and the discovery of electricity. Einstein himself described this historic movement as the decline of a "mechanical" view and the rise of a "field" view of the physical world, which helped put him on his own path to relativity, to new explanations and new mysteries.[50]

> On the wall of his study, Albert Einstein kept a portrait of Michael Faraday (1791–1867), and there could have been none more appropriate. For Faraday was the pioneer and the prophet of the grand revision that made

Einstein's work possible. The world would no longer be a Newtonian scene of . . . objects mutually attracted by the force of gravity inversely proportional to the square of the distance between them. The material world would become a tantalizing scene of subtle, pervasive "fields of force." This was just as radical as the Newtonian Revolution, and even more difficult for the lay mind to grasp. Like the Copernican Revolution in astronomy, the "Field" Revolution in physics would defy common sense and carry the pioneer scientists once again into "the mists of paradox." . . . Faraday, blessed with the amateur's naive vision, was not seduced by the revered Newton's mathematical formulae. . . . Faraday's discoveries had been the product of an unmathematical mind. But the persuasiveness of the field theory would still depend on its being given a mathematical form. This was accomplished by Faraday's admirer, James Clerk Maxwell (1831–1879), who translated Faraday's "lines" or "tubes" of force into a mathematical description of a continuous field. Just as Newton had given mathematical form to Galileo's insights, so, Einstein noted, Maxwell's equations performed a similar function for Faraday. "The formulation of these equations," Einstein . . . called "the most important event in physics since Newton's time, not only because of their wealth of content, but also because they form a pattern for a new type of law." The features of these equations would appear "in all other equations of modern physics." These equations would become a basis, too, for Einstein's own theory of relativity.[51]

The work of Edwin P. Hubble, during the 1920s, provides evidence that Einstein's general theory of relativity was having a significant impact on the development of theories of galactic evolution by contemporary astronomers. In his book *Astronomy and Cosmology,* John North has made the following observations about E. P. Hubble's work:

> Hubble's later version of his classification of nebulae (developed in 1923) provided a basis for that which is still in use. . . . By averaging the properties of . . . bright stars visible in galaxies of the great Virgo cluster, which must be of comparable distance, he found data that he could apply to still more remote galaxies. In this way Hubble built up an incomparable body of data as to galactic distances. By 1929 he had distances for eighteen galaxies and four members of the Virgo cluster. In this way Hubble provided what proved to be an essential key to a subject that for more than a decade had been theoretically prepared for it. The subject in question was

a type of cosmology that had grown, quite unforeseen, out of Einstein's general theory of relativity.[52]

> Hubble . . . was soon in possession of the best data on distances, and by 1929 he had information enough to allow him to announce a very simple law. It seemed that *the Universe of galaxies is expanding,* and that *the radial velocities of the galaxies are simply proportional to their distances from the sun.*[53]

Hubble could not have known at the time of his death in 1953 that a mighty telescope bearing his name would be lifted beyond the earth's atmosphere by a rocket, providing mankind with visions of galactic realities which would have thrilled him to the core.

All Science Is Cosmology

What conclusions can be drawn from this brief survey of the history of Western cosmologies, and the epistemologies they have spawned?

First, that the overwhelming pattern in Western thought has been to reason from assumptions, beliefs, or theories about the nature and structure of the universe to conclusions about the order and content of knowledge in all sciences. Whitehead wrote: "Abstract theory precedes the understanding of fact." Cosmology drives epistemology. We start with what we believe we know, and with what we imagine, and from there derive criteria to test our hypothesis against the world.

Second, we may conclude from this review that a relevant, viable, and useful set of conclusions about the order and content of knowledge in the field of medical science—i.e., a relevant and practical medical epistemology adequate to cope effectively with the challenges facing medical inquiry in the new millennium—will have to be founded upon a trenchant understanding of the revolutionary, leading-edge cosmological ideas of such thinkers as Darwin and Einstein. North has commented as follows on the significance of this interrelationship between and among fields of inquiry:

> It is easy to forget how deep are the potential connections between cosmology and the other sciences. To begin with theories of stellar evolution: the *parts* of the Universe are certainly in a process of change. . . . The fact

that all cosmology, all astronomy, should ideally be made to connect with other acceptable sciences—and that their histories must therefore also be linked—is not a new idea, but in an increasingly complex intellectual world the principle of division of labour tends always to force them apart. . . . Generality has always been acknowledged as one of the highest of scientific virtues.[54]

In his book *The Lives of a Cell*, Dr. Lewis Thomas has told us about the *disconnect* that he has observed in the field of medical science, pointing out that while the biological sciences have been producing a wealth of new and startling information, in the field of genetics, for example, in medicine "we still have formidable diseases, still unsolved, lacking satisfactory treatment." Thomas tells us that the word "biomedical" is being used to suggest the existence of a fruitful connectedness between the community of inquiry in biology and the research that is going on in the field of medicine, however, "There is still the conspicuous asymmetry between molecular biology and, say, the therapy of lung cancer. . . . It is possible that we are on the verge of developing a proper applied science, but it has to be said that we don't have one yet." Lewis Thomas is warning us that, in large measure because of the evident asymmetry between biology and medicine, we may be many decades away from a real breakthrough in discovering the "mechanisms of today's unsolved diseases—schizophrenia, for instance, or cancer, or stroke."[55]

His concluding advice to medical colleagues, public policy makers, and all citizens is that, given the gravity of the current situation in medicine, it is time to be open-minded, and to give careful consideration to any and all ideas "about better ways to speed things up." In this regard, it will be important to bear closely in mind the caveat offered by A. M. Taylor:

[P]opular opinion is apt to confuse science with technological success . . . so that it is only natural that, in popular imagination, technological marvels displace the wonders of science. . . . The handiwork of the craftsman is mistaken for the intellectual creation of the savant.[56]

This historical retrospective serves as a backdrop for "ideas about better ways to speed things up." If it is true that "all science is cosmology," then the science of medicine needs special scrutiny in these terms: How has it organized itself? What are the presuppositions and biases about the "nature of things" which might explain the current structures, habits, and practices of "organized medicine" in the United States? An effective and fruitful community of medical inquiry today ought to be led by thinkers—physicians—who have a keen awareness of issues in contemporary cosmology such as quantum theory and reality; and of astrophysical phenomena such as quasars, spiral galaxies, and black holes; gamma ray bursts; inflationary cosmology; red shifts as indicators of an expanding universe; X-ray astronomy; gravitational radiation; and quantum cosmology, among others. American medicine needs learned men and women in order to reform itself. It needs the stimulus of leading-edge discoveries about the nature of the universe: 100 billion stars in our galaxy, and 100 million galaxies altogether; and about all of the new knowledge flooding in behind Darwin and Einstein.

The Importance of Guessing Right

The following chapter presents an analysis of the medical "cosmos" as it has been envisioned and structured by physicians in the United States today. If it is true that "abstract theory precedes the understanding of fact," as Whitehead has observed, then it is of central importance to examine the abstract theories which currently motivate the field of medical inquiry in America, so as to assure that the understanding of the facts of clinical observation, relying as it does upon the incisiveness and validity of those theories, will be entirely appropriate, humane, and effective in achieving the highest purposes of the medical profession. Whitehead's dictum may be seen as being akin to the chicken-and-egg issue, given the fact that one must certainly have particulars in view in order to raise abstractions from them. However, this analysis would miss Whitehead's fundamental point. Another philosopher from the British Isles, Michael Polanyi, has articulated this same insight in other words:

> Scientists—that is, creative scientists—spend their lives in trying to guess right. They are sustained and guided therein by their heuristic passion. . . . Scientific discovery is more than knowledge, for it is foreknowledge of things yet unknown and at present perhaps inconceivable.[57]

The key point for American medicine today is that imagination "precedes the discovery of fact" precisely because it brings a direction to the scientific quest. Abstractions that can lead to the understanding of fact are born in the imagination and the passion of the scientist. And, it is imagination and passion that will lead the observer to focus on these particulars rather than those particulars. The intellectual leaders of contemporary American medicine have demonstrated a comfort level with their own certitudes so radical that curiosity, the driver of human imagination, is noted for its absence. The community of inquiry in medicine is therefore focused on the *wrong* set of particulars, exactly because of the prevalent deficiencies in both imagination and passion. The generation of abstract theory in medicine suffers accordingly, with the result that the field of medical inquiry today is essentially technological, geared to the improvement of invention; it is not fundamentally scientific, not geared to breakthrough and to discovery. Certitudes, although they may be false and misleading, tend to be held in a way that overwhelms the prospects for ever harboring "a foreknowledge of things unknown and at present perhaps inconceivable." The implications of these conclusions for the structure and content of clinical practice in the twenty-first century are enormous. Medicine's dominant "scheme of ideas" must undergo a radical reconstruction before the abstractions that presently drive medical education and practice can be effectively transformed.

Notes

1. A. N. Whitehead, *The Function of Reason* (Boston: Beacon Press, 1958), pp. 76–77.

2. P. Angeles, *Harper Collins Dictionary of Philosophy* (New York: Harper Perennials, 1992), p. 89.

3. D. W. Richards, "Hippocrates and History: The Arrogance of Humanism," in *Hippocrates Revisited*, ed. R. J. Bulgar (New York: MEDCOM, 1973), p. 19.

4. J. North, *Astronomy and Cosmology* (New York: W. W. Norton & Co., 1994), p. 83.

5. H. Butterfield, "Dante's View of the Universe," in *A Short History of Science* (Garden City, N.Y.: Anchor Books, n.d.), p. 9.

6. North, *Astronomy and Cosmology*, pp. 120–21.

7. D. Boorstin, *The Discoverers* (New York: Random House, 1983), p. 20.

8. North, *Astronomy and Cosmology*, p. 261.

9. Butterfield, "Dante's View of the Universe," pp. 2–5.

10. Boorstin, *The Discoverers*, pp. 341–42.

11. North, *Astronomy and Cosmology*, pp. 234–69.

12. Boorstin, *The Discoverers*, p. 71.

13. North, *Astronomy and Cosmology*, p. 248.

14. Boorstin, *The Discoverers*, pp. 338–40.

15. Ibid., p. 340.

16. Ibid., pp. 341–43.

17. H. Dale, "Harvey and the Circulation of the Blood," in *A Short History of Science*, p. 36.

18. Thomas Kuhn, *The Copernican Revolution* (Cambridge, Mass.: Harvard University Press, 1957), pp. 229–30.

19. Boorstin, *The Discoverers*, p. 305.

20. Ibid., pp. 307–308.

21. Ibid., p. 307.

22. Ibid., pp. 309–11.

23. Ibid., p. 318.

24. Kuhn, *The Copernican Revolution*, pp. 225–26.

25. Boorstin, *The Discoverers*, pp. 325–26.

26. C. D. Broad, "Bacon and the Experimental Method," in *A Short History of Science*, pp. 30–32.

27. Dale, "Harvey and the Circulation of the Blood," p. 34.

28. Boorstin, *The Discoverers*, p. 403.

29. North, *Astronomy and Cosmology*, p. 372.

30. Ibid.

31. Boorstin, *The Discoverers*, p. 378.

32. Ibid., p. 379.

33. Ibid., p. 377.

34. Ibid., pp. 376–82.

35. Ibid., pp.328–29.

36. A. N. Whitehead, *Science and the Modern World* (New York: Free Press, 1957), pp. 39–40.

37. A. N. Whitehead, *The Function of Reason* (Boston: Beacon Press, 1958), pp. 74–75.

38. F. S. Taylor, "Scientific Developments of the Early Nineteenth Century," in *A Short History of Science*, pp. 81–82.

39. Boorstin, *The Discoverers*, pp. 328–29.

40. C. F. A. Pantin, "The Origin of Species," in *A Short History of Science*, p. 94.

41. D. C. Dennett, *Darwin's Dangerous Idea* (New York: Touchstone, 1995), p. 263.

42. Ibid., pp. 19–21.

43. T. Dobzhansky, *American Biology Teacher* 35 (1973): 6–7.

44. T. Dobzhansky, *The Biological Basis of Human Freedom* (New York: Columbia University Press, 1960), pp. 27–28.

45. Ibid., pp. 118–19.

46. Ibid., pp. 87–88.

47. Ibid., pp. 104–105.

48. Dennett, *Darwin's Dangerous Idea*, p. 63.

49. North, *Astronomy and Cosmology*, p. 511.

50. Boorstin, *The Discoverers*, p. 679.

51. Ibid., pp. 679–84.

52. North, *Astronomy and Cosmology*, pp. 509–10.

53. Ibid., p. 523.

54. Ibid., pp. 597–98.

55. L. Thomas, *The Lives of a Cell* (New York: Bantam Books, 1975), pp. 134–37.

56. A. M. Taylor, *Imagination and the Growth of Science* (New York: Schocken Books, 1970), p. 1.

57. M. Polanyi, *Personal Knowledge: Towards a Post-Critical Philosophy* (Chicago: University of Chicago Press, 1958), p. 143.

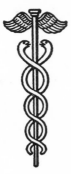

3.

The American Medical Cosmos: A Clockwork Universe

"All science is cosmology, the problem of understanding the world, ourselves, and our knowledge as part of it."
Sir Karl Popper[1]

As noted in the preceding chapter, in his essay entitled "The Function of Reason," Alfred North Whitehead defined the relationship between "cosmology" and "theories of knowledge" as being akin to that between *genus* and *species*:

> Cosmology is the effort to frame a scheme of the general character of the present stage of the universe. The cosmological scheme should present the genus, for which the special schemes of the sciences are the species.[2]

Whether the cosmological scheme—the genus—is explicit or not, it is nonetheless continuously at work in shaping the "special schemes" which determine and control the community of inquiry within a specific science, the science of medicine being one example.

Sir Karl Popper's observation that "all science is cosmology" could be modified to read: "[A]ll science is driven by an *ideology,*" with "the problem of understanding the world, our-selves and our knowledge as part of it."

The Influence of a Scheme of Ideas

In the preface to his monumental work entitled *Process and Reality, An Essay In Cosmology,* Whitehead wrote that "All constructive thought on the various topics of scientific interest is dominated by a scheme of ideas, unacknowl-edged, but no less influential in guiding the imagination."[3]

Whitehead pointed to the need for us to: "make such schemes explicit, and thereby capable of criticism and improvement." To the extent that a scheme of ideas remains inexplicit, and thereby incapable of criticism, *improvement* becomes impossible because there is no cogent means for detecting any possible error in constructive thought, or for pointing up the inadequacies lurking within a popular hypothesis or set of assumptions.

It is my contention here that contemporary medicine in the United States has unwittingly worked itself into this precise predicament. Because the scheme of ideas specific to the field of medical inquiry is wrongheaded, and because the scheme remains inexplicit, and thus immune from evalua-tion or criticism, medicine as a science has boxed itself in.

An excellent general example of this phenomenon can be taken from the Ptolemaic cosmology, which—despite being erroneous—persisted as gospel in the West for over fourteen hundred years due principally to the fact that, during those fourteen centuries, "common sense" kept getting in the way of a thoroughgoing critique of Ptolemy's incorrect cosmological scheme of ideas.

In what follows I offer some suggestions as to the unacknowledged ingredients of a scheme of ideas which might be made explicit, based upon three different examples of a *genus* related to each of three essentially different cosmological views, and of the "schemes" or *species* issuing from them.

Scheme A: Given the prevalence of a geocentric cosmological scheme (indebted to Ptolemy and Dante) as the *genus,* the "special scheme" (i.e., the *species*) controlling the community of inquiry in the field of medicine and accounting for its organization, would designate the health of the whole pop-ulation as the subject and object of medical practice. It would place the general physician in the "central position," like the earth itself. And it would have no idea of nor include any place for the concepts of "specialism" or of an explicit separation between mind and body. Under this "special scheme," all other actors in the realm of medicine would derive their knowledge and their motive force from the general physician, on whom their own position in the medical "cosmos" would be dependent. The guild structure would be predominant, and apprenticeship to a general physician would be the principal avenue of access into and of advancement within the medical field.

Scheme B: Given a cosmological scheme (genus) which, like Copernicus's concept, reversed the center of the world; a scheme that also adopted the Cartesian bifurcation of the subject matter, a human person, by separating body from mind, and which vigorously embraced the seventeenth-century notion of a clockwork universe as the foundation of its scheme of ideas; then the "special scheme" (species) dictating the shape and the bias of the medical community would undergo an analogous and equally radical alteration. The general physician would be reclassified as a second- or third-rate presence functioning at the edges of the reconstructed "cosmos"; and the status of information and data resulting from the clinical observations of generalist physicians would experience a similar fate. In this restructured medical community of inquiry, there would be little value assigned to the wealth of clinical information generated by the general or primary physician. In this new world, the abstractions and classifications controlling the collection, recording, and use of clinical information would now give primacy to the observations of "specialist" physicians who would carry on their medical practice within well-defined and narrow "secondary" and "tertiary" channels. The treatment of individual patients by "specialist" physicians would tend to emerge as the principal focus of medical practice, replacing a focus on the public health. A corollary concentration on the mechanical and technological aspects of medicine would rise above any potential interest in the more process-oriented biological and physiological subject matter of medicine. The concept of "scientific" medicine would be perversely identified with the frank channeling of medical inquiry, following the lines and crevasses of a plethora of medical "specialties" and "subspecialties." This fundamentally mechanistic, dualistic, clockwork scheme of ideas would create great difficulty for medical doctors in accepting and dealing with such biological, processive realities as germ theory, the deadly spread of infection by unwashed physicians, or the biochemical complexities involved in the nourishment and support of human metabolic systems.

Scheme C: Given a cosmological scheme (genus) which reflected the concepts of an organic, random, and expanding multiverse, the object of medical inquiry would necessarily be the human organism in all of its biochemical, biophysical, and psychosocial complexity, observed and studied in a "special scheme" (species) within the context of its unique genetic endowments and of its particular environments, with all things being considered, and nothing being omitted. This organic scheme of ideas would require the resituation of the general physician at the center of the medical universe as a "general manager"; and would require practical recognition that the principal source of insight and advancement in medical science would be the organized information drawn from the stream of clinical observations by general physicians engaged in caring for a population of patients at the primary level. "Specialism" would be reconstructed and redefined, with its place in the medical "cosmos" identified in terms of the gravitational force exerted from the central position, recaptured and reoccupied in this "special scheme" by the medical generalist.

A focus on tracking, trending, and publicly reporting clinical information which is aggregated for a sizeable population, e.g., the ten million members of an HMO such as the Kaiser Health Plan, and which has been adjusted so as to eliminate any extremes in the estimated morbidity of the specific population, would provide the source for a wealth of new insights and hypotheses, opening the pathways to achieving significant discovery and breakthrough in medical science, as contrasted with the mere continuation of technological invention. The reason for a carefully made morbidity adjustment to the data being reported for a specific population is to recognize the probability that the presence of disease in the membership of organized health plans will differ from one plan to another. In one HMO, an extraordinary number of members may have two or more chronic diseases, and the plan may therefore have a higher profile of morbidity than does the national population. A national database is readily available for use in adjusting the reporting of the clinical outcomes of care for a specific HMO to insure that a larger, or a smaller-than-average number of diabetics in the membership, for example, would not inappropriately skew the information being reported about the relative effectiveness of the medical care provided to those members, as compared with the patterns and trends of medical management in other competing HMOs.

In each of the foregoing examples of a "worldview" or cosmology (the *genus*), and of the epistemology or scheme of ideas (the *species*) flowing out of that "worldview," the ideology inhabiting the minds of medical doctors determines their behavior in making important decisions about medical practice. For the majority of American physicians today, and most especially for the physicians who dominate academic medicine, Scheme B overwhelmingly prevails. There can be no other explanation, for example, which could adequately account for the placement of surgeons firmly at the top of the contemporary medical totem. Not even an unlimited indulgence of human economic greed on the part of hospital owners and their surgical staff could explain the truly inappropriate hierarchical position held by the surgeons within the contemporary medical "cosmos." The brute fact that must be faced is that the scheme of ideas inherent in Scheme B, above, is terribly wrongheaded, and is therefore continuously misdirecting the medical community of inquiry and the practice of medicine in the United States.

It was not always so in America. Medicine began its career in the New World under the sway of the cosmological scheme highlighted in Scheme A, above—a Ptolemaic view of the universe, popularized in Dante's writings. When the Mayflower landed at Plymouth Rock, the revolutionary Copernicus had been dead for just fifty-seven years; and Vesalius for thirty-six years. Bacon was then thirty-nine years old; Galileo was thirty-six years old; Harvey was twenty-four years old, and would publish his revolutionary work on the circulation of the blood eight years later; and Descartes was just a lad of four. It would be forty-two years before Newton's birth.

At the outset of life in the seventeenth-century New World, medicine for the settlers was inevitably the direct descendent of its old European ancestor. Few physicians had emigrated to America, and in the absence of a cash economy during the early period, few immigrants could afford to return to Europe to pursue a medical education. Vesalius's textbook on anatomy was very likely the prominent reference work on a physician's bookshelf in the colonies.

At a casual level, the world according to Dante's *Divine Comedy* was undoubtedly still prevalent. Evidence of medicine's link to astrology was also present, including the ancient Greek notions about the four elements which define nature; and the four "humors" which constitute the body, any imbalance of these taken to be the source of illness among humans. Bloodletting, blistering, sweating, and purging were being practiced by physicians in colonial America.

On the other hand, the writings of Paracelsus had been around for a century, and had an impact in the New World environment in which, during the early years of adjustment, it was not difficult to believe that the causes of illness were primarily external, rather than the result of an imbalance of internal humors. The inquisitive among the colonists were surely aware of Francis Bacon's work on induction, and on the value of direct experience as the source of knowledge, as contrasted with theoretical speculation. Everyday survival in America during the early seventeenth century would lend practical reinforcement to Bacon's theoretical notion.

The few physicians who did come to America early on had adopted, out of necessity if not conviction, the patterns set out in the Oath of Hippocrates as the means of producing the additional physicians which immigrant survival in the New World would require:

> I will look upon him who shall have taught me this art even as one of my parents. I will share my substance with him, and I will supply his necessities, if he be in need. I will regard his offspring even as my own brethren and I will teach them this art, if they would learn it, without fee or covenant. I will impart this art by precept, by lecture and by every mode of teaching, not only to my own sons but to sons of him who has taught me, and to disciples bound by covenant and oath, according to the law of medicine.[4]

Apprenticeship in Early American Medicine

For most of the next three centuries, the education and training of physicians in North America was in the hands of physicians who were practicing medicine, and simultaneously taking responsibility for one or more "apprentices" who were interested in learning how to treat and care for the sick and the injured.

Except for the influence of curative practices the settlers picked up from

American "Indians," the intellectual basis for what was being taught and learned about medicine during this period of three centuries in America was, and remained, European. To the extent that textbooks or professional treatises were available to these New World physicians and their apprentices, the source of these writings was Europe: England, Holland, France, and Italy. In Europe, medicine was still emerging from the Middle Ages, when those who practiced the various medical arts, including astrology, were members of a guild. In some instances, the membership of a guild would be determined on the basis of the specific role being played in medicine. The structure and organizational principles of the European medical guilds continued to reflect their feudal origins.

The principles and the feudal structure of the medical guild were imported to the New World as a matter of course. The medical guild is a fraternity of physicians possessing all of the characteristics of free baronry, along with all of the other features of an effective feudal guild. Webster defines a guild as: "An association of men with kindred pursuits or common interests or aims for mutual aid and protection." The medical guild in America has from the outset been organized to fight off every attempt to interfere with or limit powers or turf already seized and held. The power and importance of the medical guild were accentuated in the American context by the virtual absence of universities, and by the need for physicians in practice to pass along their knowledge and skills through guild-like apprenticeship arrangements. There was simply no other available way to produce the medical manpower needed in the colonies to serve a growing population in a land whose borders were continuously expanding westward.

It is remarkable that the major features of the feudal guild have continued to characterize the fundamental relationships which medical doctors in America have maintained between and among themselves up to the present time. This enduring reality has been a significant ingredient in the complex recipe that has led American medicine to its current state of crisis. In a paper delivered at a Robert Wood Johnson Foundation workshop in January 1993, Stanford University economist Alain Enthoven made the following comment about "Guild Free Choice":

> These principles dominated the health care system in the USA until well into the 1980s, and their effects are still important today. They were

enforced by legislation (e.g., guild principles were built into all State insurance codes until the 1980s and into Title XVIII of the Social Security Act), boycotts (e.g., by doctors against hospitals contracting with HMOs), professional ostracism (e.g., from county medical societies and hospital staffs), denial of medical staff privileges, and harassment.[5]

Guild-style apprenticeship training of physicians inevitably became the standard pattern in America, throughout the seventeenth century, and through most of the eighteenth century. During this period in America, the prevailing professional opinion had been that the body of medical knowledge could be mastered by one person during one lifetime of study and practice, and it became an obligation within the physician's guild, consistent with the Oath of Hippocrates, to pass these skills and this knowledge of the medical arts on to capable men of the next generation. The American response to the major problem of producing doctors of medicine in sufficient quantity to serve a growing population evolved eventually in the form of proprietary medical schools, established by the gathering together of physicians who were already engaged in training apprentices, and who felt the need to conduct this training in a more efficient and productive way. It has been recorded that in the early part of the eighteenth century in Boston, probably America's most populous city at the time, with some 100,000 residents, there were only a half-dozen practicing physicians. The proprietary medical schools were intended to resolve this shortage.

Unlike the universities of Europe, where study of the seven liberal arts (grammar, rhetoric, logic, geometry, astronomy, arithmetic, and music) was required before a student could tackle the study of medicine, the subject matter of the American medical "schools" was generally restricted to the practical medical "arts." The principal goal of the physicians who were sponsoring the proprietary schools was to increase the number of apprentices each doctor could take on by introducing efficiencies of scale through the addition of didactic learning, designed to supplement the experiences of an on-the-job apprenticeship. Of course, as the number of apprentices per mentoring physician increased, so did the incomes of the physician sponsors.

When the proprietary medical schools began to multiply in the early 1800s, and to then spread westward as the frontier was being settled, there were no external standards applied to them, no uniformity of curriculum, no certification by an established authority. The proprietary schools, therefore, ran the gamut from what we would call "diploma mills" to the well-disciplined study of all available medical knowledge, supplemented by practical experience, and with every imaginable alternative in between. As the new century began in America, in keeping with medical guild rubrics, a "doctor" could be a man who had simply purchased a medical diploma; or one who had labored as an apprentice to a practicing physician for varying periods of time, and with varying quality in learning opportunity; or one who had completed training in a medical school (possibly with excellent curricula, or middling to very poor quality); or by a small number of men who had attended a university, in America or abroad, and who had obtained the best medical education available at the time.

> The doctor in 1860 could look back to a very considerable change in medicine. There was a decline in professional morale, as compared with the optimism of 1800, at least in the sense of medicine as an elitist calling. But the attitudes were perhaps more realistic as to the future needs for the provision of doctors and the future means of regulation. At least most practitioners now had some kind of formal education. There was a basic standard, low as it was, that most physicians met. There was a network of medical schools, poor as most of them were. . . . It was from this apparently poor but potentially fertile ground that the future structure of American medicine—and ultimately the future of specialization—was to emerge.[6]

In his 1910 report on the status of medicine in America, Abraham Flexner observed that, after nearly a hundred years of increase and expansion, near the dawn of the twentieth century, as many as 400 proprietary medical schools had been opened, and some 200 of them remained in operation, scattered across the country. They had been turning out "doctors" in significant quantities. As the result of the combined output of apprenticeship training and of the numerous proprietary medical schools in existence prior to the 1890s, by that time a surplus of physicians had been created in the United States, and the competition for patients within cities and large towns was often fierce. In fact, by the end of the nineteenth century, the doctor-to-patient ratio in America was twice that of Europe. In the space of a little over 150 years, the doctor-to-patient ratio had gone from the 6 physicians per 100,000 citizens reported in

Boston during the first half of the eighteenth century, to 200 doctors per 100,000 people in 1890, for the country as a whole.

These doctors by-and-large were general practitioners, Renaissance men in medicine whose mission it was to learn, to remember, and to teach all that there was to know about the medical arts. The fact that by 1890 one such doctor had been produced for every five hundred persons in the United States explains our perception that there was a "Doc Adams" in every frontier town in the country. During the last half of the nineteenth century, there were so many doctors competing for patients in the major population centers of America that a number of them picked up and headed west, heeding the famous advice Horace Greeley offered to the unemployed in New York City during the 1850s.

Most of these doctors were practicing a second or third-rate version of European medicine and were at least a half-century behind the knowledge base of the average practicing physician in Europe. During this period, the medical professors of European universities viewed American medical practices and educational standards as woefully inferior to those prevalent on the continent or in the British Isles, and they were not wrong.

Academic Medicine in Europe

During this same period, Europe was undergoing intellectual ferment as the centuries-old certitudes of Ptolemaic cosmology were being called into serious question. The theories of Copernicus were attracting attention, if not adherents, and Professor Galileo had pointed his telescope toward the heavens, and talked about his through-the-lens experiences. The pattern in Europe, including the British Isles, reflected an increasing respect for and reliance upon the academic training of physicians, usually in universities, with major emphasis on didactic learning in the liberal arts as a foundation for medical education. Such lesser medical lights as surgeons and apothecaries continued to be trained in apprenticeships in Europe, however by the middle of the eighteenth century, many of the physicians in "general practice" had received medical degrees as the result of completing the prescribed course of study in a university. By this time, the cosmological theories of René Descartes had infiltrated the medical curricula throughout Europe, and the influences of Newton's crystallizing work were evident everywhere.

In the last quarter of the nineteenth century, it was still the case that Americans interested in studying medicine at the leading edge of medical knowledge would have to go abroad to do so. And before being accepted at an established European university, they would have to prepare themselves in the seven liberal arts, thereby gaining an academic background that was almost totally lacking among doctors in eighteenth- and nineteenth-century America.

The Seductive Mechanical Model

In Europe, the seventeenth century notion of a "clockwork universe" was ultimately articulated with consummate clarity by Sir Isaac Newton. Daniel Boorstin recalls in the *Discoverers* the metaphor that Nicole d'Oresme had written in the fourteenth century: "a clockwork universe, God the perfect clockmaker!" and links it to the cosmological schemes formulated by Johannes Kepler and by René Descartes:

> This metaphor guided and inspired scientists like the great astronomer Johannes Kepler. "My aim," he observed in 1605, "*is to show that the celestial machine is to be likened not to a divine organism but rather to a clockwork*" (emphasis added). And Descartes, too, the philosopher-mathematician, made the clock his prototypical machine. His doctrine of dualism—that mind and body operated independently—was explained in a famous clock metaphor. Suppose there are two clocks, Descartes's Dutch disciple [Arnold] Geulinex suggested, both of which keep perfect time. When one points to the hour, the other always strikes. If you did not know about their machinery and how they were made, you might mistakenly assume that the movements of the one caused the other to strike. This is the way both the mind and the body function. God the Clockmaker created each quite independently of the other, then wound up both of them and set them going so they are in perfect harmony. When I decide to lift my arm, I may think that my mind is acting on my body. But really both move independently, each a part of God's perfectly harmonized clockwork.[7]

Unable to discover a rational methodology for dealing with the "mind/ body" problem, Descartes determined that it would be intellectually acceptable to separate these aspects of reality, to ignore the fluency of things, and to concentrate on the enduring aspects of human experience. The objects, the "things" in nature have thereby become the principal focus of modern medical inquiry; and medicine has tended to relegate to the back burner the more processive elements, the complex "events" of nature, and of human being.

Borelli's initiation of the field of *iatrophysics* pushed medicine firmly in the direction of Descartes and Newton, and away from the more processive, less mechanistic notions of such Enlightenment thinkers as Leibniz or Spinoza. Borelli demonstrated that the human body had the same qualities and movements as all other physical things. Boorstin describes Borelli's beliefs as follows:

> Movements of the limbs, in lifting, walking, running, jumping, and skating . . . followed the laws of physics. . . . [T]hese same physical laws [apply] to the movements of muscles and the heart, the circulation of the blood, and the process of respiration.[8]

Herbert Butterfield, professor of modern history at Cambridge, has made the following observation about the Cartesian and Newtonian bias of seventeenth-century thought:

> [T]he whole mechanistic trend of the seventeenth-century scientific movement produced the result that the mechanical explanations were the things to look for, even in subjects like biology where we now know that purely mechanical explanations are insufficient.[9]

A quotation from E. A. Burtt's work, *The Metaphysical Foundations of Modern Physical Science,* provides additional underpinning for the conclusions being drawn in this volume about the impact of a mechanistic metaphysics on medical science:

> It was of the greatest consequence for succeeding thought that now the great Newton's authority was squarely behind that view of the cosmos which saw in man a puny, irrelevant spectator . . . of the vast mathematical system whose regular motions according to mechanical principles constituted the world of nature . . . a world hard, cold, colourless, silent and dead —a world of quantity, a world of mathematically computable motions in

mechanical regularity. . . . In Newton, the Cartesian metaphysics, ambiguously interpreted and stripped of its distinctive claim for serious philosophical consideration, finally overthrew Aristotelianism, and became the predominant world-view of modern time.[10]

In his essay entitled *On the Limitations of Modern Medicine,* Thomas McKeown wrote:

The approach to biology and medicine established during the seventeenth century was an engineering one based on a physical model. Nature was conceived in mechanistic terms, which led in biology to the idea that a living organism could be regarded as a machine which might be taken apart and reassembled if its structure and function were fully understood. In medicine, the same concept led further to the belief that an understanding of disease processes and of the body's response to them would make it possible to intervene therapeutically, mainly by physical (surgical), chemical, or electrical methods.[11]

Rick J. Carlson, in his book *The End of Medicine,* reached the following conclusions about the impact on medicine of seventeenth-century mechanistic and dualistic beliefs:

The Cartesian thesis that mind and matter were divisible drove a wedge between the mind and the body that persists in medicine today despite its repudiation everywhere else. . . . As a way of looking at the world, it was seized by medicine as a way of organizing its endeavor . . . a shaman was not needed to tinker with a machine; what was needed was a mechanic. The class of shamans could now be replaced by a class of mechanics. . . . The doctor had emerged, *but a cohesive theoretical framework for medicine had not* [emphasis added]. The idea of the body as a machine is elegant to the biologist and highly explanatory. However, in medicine's hands it was perverted in practice. To think of man as a machine does aid us in understanding something about bodily function and about man's role in the universe, but it does not follow that treating the body as a machine will heal it. But medicine appropriated the idea as the premise for its practice.[12]

Mechanism Predominates

The new mechanistic cosmology had finally achieved primacy in Europe's centers of learning. The great European universities in Padua, Prague, and Paris had had two centuries or more of history, tradition, and intellectual ferment underlying the adoption of the "clockwork universe" as the prevailing cosmological view of the world. The New World, on the other hand, was for a long time totally lacking in academies of higher learning, and therefore without the opportunities a scholarly community of inquiry could provide for professional students of medicine; and without an effective means to overcome their weak and shaky professional reputation, at home and abroad.

In nineteenth-century America, as the apprenticeship training of doctors had become more organized, formalized, and widespread, and as a handful of university-based medical faculties emerged, the scheme of ideas held by American doctors eventually began to reflect the transition that had taken place much earlier throughout Europe: away from the worldview depicted by Dante, Ptolemaic to its roots, and toward the earth-moving cosmology of the Copernican Revolution, influenced by the work of Galileo, and bound to a purely mechanistic concept of nature through the genius of René Descartes.

During the final years of the nineteenth century and the early years of the twentieth, the American medical guild began formally embracing as its own the erroneous cosmological scheme developed in seventeenth-century Europe; and began adopting along with it the equally erroneous theories of knowledge spawned by the mechanistic and dualistic cosmology of a "clockwork universe." As the twentieth century was beginning, the ideology of the American medical guild was exhibiting the *genus* of a clockwork cosmology, and the *species* of a thoroughly mechanistic and dualistic scheme of ideas, an importation of European ideas which by then were at least three centuries old.

With the dawn of the twentieth century, three principal convergent forces were of major significance in shaping the American medical structure currently in place, as another new century looms on the horizon:

1. American doctors shared a widespread belief that their education, experience, and medical practice were inferior in comparison with their European counterparts; and shared a recognition that they were the victims

of vicious satiric humor, and of patient complaints about the competence and quality of their medicine.

2. The large surplus of physicians in general practice in the United States at the time created an unusually fertile ground for the development of "specialty" education in medicine, on a scale which has never been undertaken in Europe.

3. A cascade of discoveries and information directly affecting the art of medicine occurred, nourished most particularly by Pasteur's reporting of his use of the microscope to observe the microcosmos; and by Darwin's *Origin of Species* in 1859, the same year in which Sigmund Freud presented his first major work in psychoanalysis.

The American medical guild was now presented with an unprecedented opportunity, created by this convergence of forces, which could enable it to overcome the widespread reputation, and its own belief, that its medical education and medical practices were far inferior to European medicine; which could enable the profession to cope with the explosion of information about the human species already building up at the turn of the century; and which could enable specialty-trained physicians to wrest control of the medical guild from the generalists, and to dominate the professional guild for the foreseeable future.

Whereas William Harvey's discovery of the circulatory system had involved a phenomenon which humans share with other mammals, the information which now began to pour forth from the work of Pasteur, Darwin, and Freud, among others, applied uniquely to human beings. Brand new fields of inquiry were being introduced into the field of medicine. The long list of "ologies" which define contemporary medicine have their origins within this nineteenth-century watershed of new insight into the human species and the world it inhabits. New World medicine did not, however, adjust its prevailing scheme of ideas to reflect the organic, random, and processive cosmological presuppositions of Pasteur and Darwin. On the contrary, American medicine has adhered quite firmly to the erroneous cosmology of the clockwork universe. In his essay entitled *Scientific Developments of the Early Nineteenth Century*, F. Sherwood Taylor, the director of the Science Museum in South Kensington, London, made the following observations:

We [had] seen . . . in the years 1800–1840 very great discoveries in most of the sciences. . . . the biological sciences had little effect upon medicine at this period, the chief advances of which arose from clinical observation or experiment. [Edward] Jenner's discovery of vaccination was the result of keen observation, not of medical theory.[13]

Once the watershed had broken, however, it became evident that it would be impossible to contain the entirety of medical knowledge within the mind of a single physician at any given point in time. Surely, the generalist physician would not be able to master all of the new knowledge now flooding in. Common sense would require specialization, and dictate the reorganization of medical knowledge into channels that would, inevitably, be both deeper and more narrow. The hydra-head of medical specialization was becoming visible, and the study and practice of medicine would thus undergo a radical transformation.

The early reaction of the medical fraternity in America to the explosion of biological information which followed Darwin's trenchant work was succinctly described by Julius Richmond, M.D., who served as chairman of the Department of Pediatrics at upstate Medical Center in Syracuse, New York: "Concomitant with the growth of scientific knowledge . . . was the emergence of specialization." Dr. Richmond made the following observations about the changes that occurred in the United States during this period:

At the turn of the century, scientific advances were beginning to have a significant impact on medical education and medical care. . . . These scientific developments presented medicine with certain alternatives. First, medical education could go on, as it had in the nineteenth century, training large numbers of physicians through a network of medical schools, many of which were privately owned and managed. This system had produced a favorable physician-population ratio; the relatively large numbers of physicians assured a reasonable distribution to rural as well as urban areas. Medical education was mainly in the hands of practitioners of medicine and reflected the struggles and rivalries of individuals and groups. For example, if a resourceful and able physician was dissatisfied with his fate in one school, he could go off and organize one of his own—and he often did. The history of this period is replete with colorful figures who were itinerants in medical education and who established a string of medical schools in the course of their migrations. . . . The second alternative, attempting to improve rapidly all the existing schools, did not seem realistic in terms of available scientific personnel and other resources. The third alternative, the introduction of standards and accrediting processes which would make it impossible for many of these schools to survive, gradually evolved. The catalyst for this development was the Flexner Report of 1910, which presents a detailed account of the state of medical education and practice during the first decade of this century.[14]

Looking back to the period just prior to the landing of the settlers at Plymouth Rock, the European medical "tree of knowledge" had displayed no more than ten branches. According to the *Medical Family Tree*, an elaborate and detailed map of European and American medicine published in Germany in 1989 by Rolf Winau and Peter von Burtkowski, the branches of medical "specialization" in the West, from the Middle Ages until 1623, included the following, in rough chronological order:

1.	Surgery	(1280s)
2.	Obstetrics & Gynecology	(1500s)
3.	Pediatrics	(1500s)
4.	Anatomy	(1530s)
5.	Embryology	(1550s)
6.	Ophthalmology	(1550s)
7.	Dentistry	(1560s)
8.	Dermatology	(1580s)
9.	Venereology	(1580s)
10.	Physiology	(1580s)

In the intervening two and a half centuries between the arrival of the Mayflower in America and Darwin's publication of his *Origin of Species*, the European medical tree of knowledge, nourished by the attractiveness and the spreading influence of the Cartesian mechanistic cosmology, sprouted an additional ten branches:

1.	Histology	(1650s)
2.	Neurology	(1650s)

3.	Eye-Nose-Throat	(1680s)
4.	Orthopaedics	(1700)
5.	Forensic Medicine	(1700)
6.	Pathology	(1750)
7.	Psychiatry	(1750s)
8.	Nephrology	(1800)
9.	Urology	(1806)
10.	Oncology	(1838)

In the hundred and twenty-odd years since Darwin's work caused a watershed of human biological information to burst on the scene, and with its roots remaining firmly in the fertile mechanistic scheme of ideas inherited from René Descartes, the medical family tree realized a growth of over 400 percent in the number of discreet medical "specialties," with the result that more than sixty additional branches now appear on the medical tree of knowledge. The principal conclusions to be noted from these irreducible facts are: (1) that during a period of a little over a hundred years, the number of medical "specialties" has exploded to more than four times the pre-Darwinian number; and, (2) nearly 35 percent of the newly added "specialties" are surgical. It is also noteworthy that the name of no American physician appears in the aforementioned *Medical Family Tree* as the founder of an "ology" until well into the first half of the twentieth century.

Despite the central importance of Darwin's opening of science to a wealth of new human information, and despite the vibrant notion of organism that formed the heart of his theory, the explosion of medical specialties that occurred during the present century reflects neither a fundamental shift in medicine's embrace of a seventeenth-century medical cosmology, nor a shift in the theories of knowledge that continue to dominate contemporary academic medicine. On the contrary, the scheme of ideas guiding the imagination of American medicine has continued to display the specific spectrum of biases that flow from a mechanistic and dualistic view of the universe in general and of the human organism in particular.

American medicine was, however, forced to cope with a radical new departure in the content and organization of medical knowledge, and with equally radical changes in the scale and the pecking order of the newly emerging and rapidly expanding medical hierarchy. The growth of specialization, which was fostered by the Council on Medical Education of the American Medical Association, the medical guild's national lobby; and by Abraham Flexner, beginning during the first ten or fifteen years of this century, has served to cement what Alfred North Whitehead identified as the bifurcation of nature, which has misguided medical inquiry in this country ever since, and which can be seen as continuing to mislead American medical inquiry, education and practice as the twentieth century draws to a close.

An Unbelievable Conception

The fatal flaw within the scheme of ideas that has dominated American medicine during the past one hundred years is a flaw directly attributable to the great Frenchman, René Descartes: the subject and the object of modern medical inquiry have been understood primarily in mechanistic and dualistic terms. Descartes' inability to solve the mind-body problem in his quest for a complete, "rational" understanding of the human being led him to conclude that it was intellectually acceptable to recognize the separateness of the substantive and the processive aspects of nature, and to proceed to engage in physical science on this basis. The resulting bifurcation of object and event, thing and process, permanence and fluency, body and mind may be seen as the root cause of the trouble with the scheme of ideas forming the intellectual base of American medicine today.

Consider Whitehead's critique of the impact of Cartesian cosmology on what we like to call the "modern" world:

> Nature is a dull affair, soundless, scentless, colourless; merely the hurrying of material, endlessly, meaninglessly. However you disguise it, this is the practical outcome of the characteristic scientific philosophy which closed the seventeenth century. In the first place, we must note its astounding efficiency as a system of concepts for the organization of scientific research. In this respect, it is fully worthy of the genius of the century which produced it. It has held its own as the guiding principle of scientific studies ever since. It is still reigning. Every university in the world organizes itself in accordance with it. No alternative system of organizing the pursuit of scientific truth has been suggested. It is not only reigning, but it is without a rival. *And yet—it is quite unbelievable. This conception of the universe is surely*

framed in terms of high abstractions, and the paradox only arises because we have mistaken our abstraction for concrete realities . . . this juggling with abstractions can never overcome the inherent confusion introduced by the ascription of misplaced concreteness to the scientific scheme of the seventeenth century.[15] (Emphasis added)

Whitehead turned to poetry for an illustration of this point:

> Abide with me.
> Fast falls the eventide.[16]

With seven words, the poet has captured a central insight, an insight of profound importance to the future directions of American medicine: human experience and existence include both stable and fleeting aspects. History demonstrates that human thinking generally has found far more comfort dealing with the stable aspects of experience, and has tended to have significant difficulty with, or to simply ignore the more processive, changing, fleeting aspects. Within the broad spectrum of scientific inquiry, perhaps nowhere else has this been more true than in the field of medicine.

As Whitehead states, the two lines of the poem "cannot be torn apart"[17] without a resulting distortion in our understanding of the subject matter at hand. Medical science has perceived the object of its study—the human body—as being substantial in nature, and as being most analogous to a machine. This fundamentally erroneous perception has been the most significant cause of the repeated instances of arrogance and blindness on the part of physicians when they have been confronted with matters of irreducible fact related to the more processive aspects of the human body, and of nature. There is an impressive and consistent history of attempts in medicine to fit distinct facts of biological science into a mechanistic scheme of ideas, each instance pointing anew to the harsh conclusion that "modern" medicine behaves in ways that are, if not unscientific, fundamentally nonscientific.

Persistent Resistance to Asepsis

A concrete example of this pattern, drawn from the 1840s and noted by John Robbins, recipient of the 1994 Rachel Carson Award for his writings, and the author of *Reclaiming Our Health,* has to do with a deep-seated pattern of physician aversion to embracing aseptic procedures, hand washing in particular:

> In the middle of the nineteenth century, a young Hungarian-born obstetrician by the name of Ignaz Phillip Semmelweis was delivering babies in a famous Viennese hospital. Women coming to give birth here were sent to one of the hospital's two sections—the First Clinic, where obstetricians prevailed and medical students received training; or the Second Clinic, staffed entirely by midwives. Noticing that women were literally begging to be admitted to the Second Clinic, Semmelweis began to look carefully at the autopsy records from the two sections. . . . What he discovered was that the death rate from puerperal [childbed] fever for women in the doctors' wards was more than four times higher than for women under the midwives' jurisdiction. Semmelweis, like the other doctors of his time, had no idea that germs could cause disease. . . . But in a moment of inspiration he decreed that the medical students handling deliveries on his ward should wash their hands in a chlorine solution after dissecting corpses, and after each examination of a woman in the ward. . . . The results were outstanding. Before the hand washing, one out of every eight women giving birth in the First Clinic had died of puerperal fever. But now the death rate dropped almost immediately to less than 1 in 100. What do you think the reaction was when Semmelweis published the records of this spectacular success? . . . Orthodox obstetricians virtually declared war on the poor man, battering and insulting him at every opportunity. He was hounded from Vienna, and eventually driven insane by the relentless attacks. He died without ever knowing that his views would eventually triumph, and that thanks to his discoveries, puerperal fever would nearly disappear. Why were such spectacular results dismissed by the medical establishment of the day? . . . [T]he finger was being pointed at obstetricians, who found it inconceivable that their own hands might be spreading the fatal infection. . . . In the United States, the chief advocate of Semmelweis's ideas was the illustrious Oliver Wendell Holmes, M.D. In April 1843, Holmes published an article titled "The Contagiousness of Puerperal Fever" in what was then known as the *New England Quarterly Journal of Medicine.* One of the country's leading obstetricians, Dr. Hugh L. Hodge, took immediate offense, and shot back with an article of his own, oppositionally titled "The Non-Contagious Character of Puerperal Fever." The very idea was preposterous, he countered, that physicians could "ever convey, in any possible

manner, [anything as] destructive as puerperal fever." It was "cruel, very cruel," he went on, to suggest to a woman that her trusted doctor could possibly bring the deadly contagion. "It is far more humane," he explained, in a burst of chivalry, "to keep her happy in ignorance of danger." At this point, another prominent obstetrician, Dr. Charles D. Meigs, leapt into the fray, accusing Holmes of "propagating a vile, demoralizing superstition." It was impossible for doctor's hands to spread disease, he declared, because doctors were gentlemen. Due to the refusal of the medical establishment to openly consider the evidence advanced by Semmelweis and Holmes, hundreds of thousands of women continued to die needlessly.[18]

With an arrogance identical to that of the Inquisitors who ridiculed the scientific discoveries of Galileo, the haughty adversaries of hand washing by obstetricians were demonstrating that, in nineteenth century Boston, the authority of the established medical guild would hold sway over the absolute correctness of the judgments of doctors like Semmelweis and Holmes about what would best protect the lives of their female patients during childbirth. The free medical baronry asserted that authority would prevail over experience; unexamined certitudes would be taken as more persuasive than scientific demonstration; and any physician colleague who dared to rebel would be hounded out of the professorship, and be banished from the medical guild on grounds of treason, no matter what the murderous consequences for childbearing women. Professor Holmes subsequently had this to say about the attitudes of his medical colleagues: "throw out wine . . . and the vapors which produce the miracle of anaesthesia, and I firmly believe that if the whole *materia medica,* as now used, could be sunk to the bottom of the sea, it would be all the better for mankind—and all the worse for the fishes."[19]

Jurgen Thorwald, the author of *The Century of the Surgeon,* started life as Heinz Bongartz. He adopted Thorwald as a pseudonym, and in 1949, after publishing his first few books as Jurgen Thorwald, he made it his legal name. He started college as a medical student, later switching to philology; however, his books reflect continuing interest in the field of medicine. In writing about the evolution of surgical practice in the West, Thorwald imagined the response that a dedicated, concerned and competent medical doctor ought to have had to Semmelweis's discoveries:

That is the fact. I who had been a witness of the discovery of anesthesia, who thought myself one of the most progressive-minded young doctors of my generation—I did not grasp the significance . . . of Semmelweis's discovery of "contact infection." Yet that discovery might then and there [have] spelled the end of the whole murderous breed of infectious diseases of surgical wounds—pyemia, erysipelas, tetanus, and wound fever—from the operating rooms of the world. I was no more intelligent than the famous professors of medicine in Europe who were damning and mocking young Semmelweis, or filing away his reports as of no importance. . . . Today that may seem incomprehensible. But it demonstrates the extent to which all of us, with very few exceptions, are slaves of established notions, and how difficult it is for us to accept anything new—all the more difficult when the new thing appears too simple possibly to be the solution to complicated problems.[20]

By the last quarter of the nineteenth century, the medical schools at Harvard and Johns Hopkins were well established as oases of European medicine in America—the former more on the British model, and the latter very explicitly on the German model. In early 1890, nearly a half-century after Holmes's battle over hand washing at Harvard Medical College, and five years before Pasteur's death, William Stewart Halsted, professor of surgery at the newly established Johns Hopkins Medical School, caused the Goodyear Rubber Company to produce a rubber glove which could be sterilized by boiling, and which was thin enough not to interfere with the surgeon's "feel" during an operation. The gloves were developed because a surgical nurse, eventually married to Halsted, had developed a debilitating skin condition on her hands from washing them in carbolic acid, in accordance with the procedures of "Listerism." If the new protective gloves worked for Caroline Hampton, she would be able to remain in Baltimore as a surgical nurse. If they did not result in curing her eczema, Halsted would almost certainly be separated from the woman whom he married in June of 1890. Although Caroline wore the new surgical gloves during all operations from then on, Halsted wore them during certain procedures, and sometimes removed them during a procedure, so as to assure himself the unimpeded "feel" which many surgeons believed the gloves interfered with. Seven more years passed until, in 1897, Halsted made the wearing of the rubber surgical gloves mandatory for all participants in all surgical procedures at Johns Hopkins. Thorwald quotes Halsted as follows:

> You cannot expect people who have all their lives not cleaned their hands and instruments, and who have worn their operating jackets until these were stiff with blood and pus, to suddenly begin believing in the wicked bacteria. Most of our medical men have never peered into a microscope. To put antisepsis across, a new generation of surgeons is needed. And it may well be that Lister is only the precursor.[21]

In Holmes's time, the word *bacteriology* did not exist. Prior to the contributions of Pasteur, Lister, and Koch, nothing was known about bacteria. In fact, as late as 1871, Joseph Lister was using the word ferments in his writings describing the presence of bacteria. But once Pasteur had published his brilliant paper "Memorandum on the Minute Organic Bodies that Exist in the Atmosphere" in 1862, the doctrine of spontaneous generation was put to death, and the facts forced the realization that microscopic organisms in the environment were the source of infection.

The challenges posed for doctors of medicine by Pasteur's discoveries have been truly profound. For surgeons, who in the European setting have never been accepted as being true physicians, the challenges have stirred deep resentment and continuous controversy, right up to the present. Justine Davis Randers-Pherson, who graduated from the Sorbonne in 1929 and earned a master's degree at Radcliffe in 1932, and who worked at the National Library of Medicine in Washington, D.C., until 1958, has written as follows about the impact of these nineteenth-century discoveries on surgeons:

> Consider that after three thousand static years, the surgeons of the nineteenth century had been abruptly hurtled into the shining new world of asepsis. . . . It had not yet occurred to them that germs could be excluded during the course of operations: germs could be killed—that was the triumph. . . . Because of this oversimplification, the surgeons were blissfully unaware of their blunders, failing to see the glaring inconsistencies.[22]

The following quotation from her book *The Surgeon's Glove* captures some of the feelings of puzzlement, frustration and anger which afflicted many sur-

geons in America during the late years of the nineteenth century and the first
part of the twentieth century:

> Robert I. Morris made . . . a colorful speech . . . to the surgical section of
> the New York Academy of Medicine, in which he deplored the decadence
> which he saw in American surgery, blaming it on the adoption of rubber
> gloves. The tirade was delivered in 1907, by which time most surgeons had
> accepted them. "We put on gloves for a boxing match with the patient's
> vitality. . . . The use of rubber gloves made it necessary to use such long
> incisions that we could work by sight. . . . Long incisions are used for
> killing bears. . . . The coming generation of surgeons brought up on
> rubber gloves will not do the wizardlike work that was done by
> older operators.[23]

At Johns Hopkins, W. S. Halsted had been completely dedicated to
using the antiseptic procedures known as "Listerism" in his operating room,
and, as noted, in 1897 he finally began requiring the use of the rubber gloves
which he had asked Goodyear to produce, this time for the expressed purpose
of protecting his surgical patients from iatrogenic illness and nosocomial
infection. (An *iatrogenic* illness is one that is caused by the doctor or other
hospital attendants under the supervision of the physician, as the result of
their medical interventions with a patient. The word is derived from the
Greek word for physician [*iatro*] and the Latin word for cause [*genesis*]. A
nosocomial infection is a hospital-acquired infection, neither present nor
incubating prior to the patient being admitted to the hospital, but usually
occurring within seventy-two hours after admission. The word is derived
from the Greek words *nosos* [disease] and *komeion* [to take care of].) The operating surgeon and all assistants now began to use the gloves in an effort to
reduce the incidence of acute infection resulting from surgery. Halsted began
reporting spectacular results in the reduction of infection and of mortality. In
the same year, 1897, at Roosevelt Hospital in New York, a surgeon named
Charles McBurney made the same decision:

> The real source of infection of a wound deliberately made by a careful sur-
> geon who uses perfect materials and handles them perfectly is to be sought
> either in the skin of the patient or in the hands of those directly concerned
> in the operation. . . . Why then not cover the hands with a material that

can be boiled? . . . it was only in April last (i.e., 1897) that I determined to use them systematically. I and my assistants used them. But in the course of three months there were several imperfect wounds. I then made up my mind that my system was not complete, for while my first assistant and I both wore gloves, my other assistants who handled instruments, ligatures, etc., did not. Since the middle of October . . . I and all my assistants have worn rubber gloves at every operation of every kind. . . . No change of methods has ever been so completely and delightfully satisfactory.[24]

The obstetric wards which physicians such as Semmelweis and Holmes had pioneered were separate facilities that came to be known as "lying-in" hospitals. These hospitals had emerged particularly in large cities, and the practice was to admit pregnant women to the "lying-in" hospital well before their due date, and to keep them in bed for a week to ten days beyond the birth of their baby. Busy OB-GYNs and general practitioners would visit these women daily, either under a global fee, or based on a per-visit charge. Doctors would come over from the general hospital where they may have been performing or assisting in a surgery; or, in some cases, where they had been performing or assisting with an autopsy.

As the direct result of their interventions with their "lying-in" patients, women and their babies were dropping like flies. The popular name for these hospitals became the "death houses." The information about the iatrogenic disasters that were occurring around the turn of the century in the many "lying-in" hospitals in large metropolitan areas became so widespread that many general physicians began advising their pregnant patients to have their babies at home, and this pattern persisted well into the 1930s. The obstinate refusal of reputable American surgeons to wash their hands prior to examining and treating their pregnant and postpartum patients was rooted in the astounding ignorance and arrogance of these doctors, despite the indisputable scientific evidence and insight that Joseph Lister, Ignaz Semmelweis, Louis Pasteur, and others had provided.

This indisputable slice of American medical history was clearly in evidence less than a century ago. It provides sufficient proof of the conclusion that, at the dawning of the twentieth century, thirty-eight years after the death of Louis Pasteur, the men at the helm of American medicine—those who directed its hospitals, dictated the content of medical education and controlled the gateway to guild membership—were arguing against the existence of the microcosmos, and about the relevance of germ theory for the practice of medicine. These physicians most assuredly would not merit having the title of "scientist" assigned to them.

In the November/December 1996 issue of *Health* magazine, Katherine Griffin published an article, entitled "They Should Have Washed Their Hands," which indicates how little this predominant medical mindset has changed. Griffin states: "*More Americans die from hospital infections every year than from car wrecks and homicides combined. Many of these tragedies could be avoided—if only nurses and doctors would clean up their act. . . . After heart disease, stroke and cancer, hospital-acquired infections are the nation's next biggest cause of death*" (emphasis added). Griffin quotes William Jarvis, chief of investigation and prevention for the Centers for Disease Control and Prevention's (CDC's) Hospital Infections Program, as saying: "The proportion (of hospital-acquired infections) that leads to death is probably increasing." Griffin goes on to say:

> Study after study has concluded that hospital workers are shockingly lax about keeping their hands clean. Hand washing has been the first line of defense against hospital infections since 1847, when an Austrian doctor named Ignaz Semmelweis first made doctors aware that they were infecting their own patients. When he bucked convention by getting doctors to wash up after dissecting cadavers, the change cut maternity ward deaths by more than 90 percent. Hospital workers today are supposed to wash their hands vigorously for two minutes before starting each shift and then for ten to fifteen seconds before every contact with a patient, even if they're going to put on surgical gloves. By now you'd think the practice would have become second nature. But it hasn't. "Experts in infection control coax, cajole, threaten and plead," railed a recent editorial in the *New England Journal of Medicine*, "and still their colleagues neglect to wash their hands." In a comprehensive review of 37 studies on hand washing, epidemiologist Elaine Larson of the Georgetown University School of Nursing found that doctors and nurses typically washed their hands only 40 percent of the time. That figure held true even in intensive care units, with their mix of highly vulnerable patients and virulent bugs. And in some of these studies the health care workers knew they were being watched. . . . This isn't rocket science . . . it's a basic concept we teach kids. But somehow people don't really believe that dirty hands can be a vehicle for infection.[25]

The CDC estimates that, each year in the United States, more than two million patients develop nosocomial infections during, and as a direct result of, their admission to an acute-care hospital. In 1970, CDC inaugurated the National Nosocomial Infection Surveillance System (NNIS) to track and report on the incidence of these infections.

The CDC reports that two million patients who are admitted to an acute-care hospital in the United States during any given year will develop such a nosocomial infection concludes that, for at least 80,000 of these unfortunate patients, this infection will either directly cause their death, or else be a major factor contributing to it.

The federal agency responsible for tracking and reporting to the public on the leading causes of death in the nation is not the CDC, but the National Center for Health Statistics (NCHS), a unit of the Public Health Service which is part of the Department of Health and Human Services (HHS). NCHS regularly publishes the *Atlas of United States Mortality.* A recent edition of the *Atlas,* released on April 17, 1997, presents the eighteen leading causes of death in the United States. The edition *does not include* a category for nosocomial infections. If the *Atlas* did include this category, the deaths caused by these infections, as currently reported by the CDC, would place nosocomial infections in the top five nonaccidental causes of death in America. To put this fact in sharper perspective, deaths now reported by the CDC as being caused by nosocomial infections are *two and a half times* the number of deaths caused annually by HIV infection. HIV/AIDS infection is now among the top ten causes of death in the nation, but is not among the top five.

Why would the NCHS fail to track and report on nosocomial infections, given the indisputable fact that they are a leading cause of death for Americans? Here is what that federal agency has to say in response to this question:

> NCHS does not collect data on nosocomial infections, however, the data are available from the Centers for Disease Control and Prevention, National Center for Infectious Diseases.[26]

The CDC has, in turn, made the following statement about its role in tracking and reporting the incidence of nosocomial infections: "NNIS is the only source of national surveillance data on nosocomial infections in the United States."[27]

These two statements constitute a perceived politically correct way for federal agencies to announce to the public that a definitive and bright line has been drawn in order to insure the elimination from the *Atlas* of one category of the *Vital and Health Statistics* which the NCHS gathers and reports for the benefit of the nation: nosocomial infections. The statements by the NCHS and the CDC are also an indication that a public servant dare not cross that definitive and bright line. Can there be any doubt that this barrier to the normal reporting of vital mortality information to the society by the NCHS has been erected at the behest of the American medical guild, with the help of its friends in the U.S. Congress?

Consider the fact that the only means of tracking hospital death rates in general was brought to an end in 1995 when federal regulators ceased requiring these reports from hospitals participating in the Medicare and Medicaid programs. The medical community lobbied the Congress strongly and effectively to force federal agencies to cease and desist the tracking and reporting of general hospital death rates.

How has CDC's Hospital Infections Program been managing its delegated responsibility to track and report on nosocomial infections, which cause at least 80,000 deaths each year? In 1984, fourteen years after the NNIS system was launched, the CDC reported that a total of 51 out of 6,375 acute-care hospitals in the United States were regularly reporting nosocomial infections. Ten years after that, by 1994, the CDC reported that the number of acute-care hospitals reporting under NNIS had grown to 180. The latest NNIS report, released in May 1997, indicates that 257 acute-care hospitals were actively participating in the NNIS system. This radical underreporting, with less than 4 percent of acute-care hospitals cooperating with the NNIS system, prevails despite the hard fact that, each and every year, nosocomial infections represent one of the five leading causes of death for American citizens. It is only logical to conclude that the 257 voluntarily cooperating hospitals are among the best facilities at controlling the incidence of nosocomial infections. Since the data submitted by these hospitals is being extrapolated by CDC to arrive at the estimate of two million nosocomial infection cases per year, it would be equally logical to conclude that the actual incidence of these infections occurring in U.S. hospitals is being understated in CDC reports, and that there are more than two million nosocomial infections, and more than 80,000 deaths each year resulting from these infections.

It is interesting to note that between 1970 and the present the number of acute-care hospitals in the nation has *increased* to over seven thousand, thus the total number of facilities that currently provide NNIS reports to the CDC equates to roughly one-third of the hospitals that have been *added* to the national inventory since the NNIS program began. It is equally noteworthy that the CDC's policy is to not release to the public the identity of the hospitals that do participate in the NNIS system.

The CDC's Hospital Infections Program estimates that the annual cost of caring for the over two million nosocomial infections exceeds $3.5 billion, and suggests that at least one-third, and perhaps one-half of these infections:

> Can be prevented by well-organized infection control programs, yet only 6 percent to 9 percent are actually prevented. . . . Since 1980, nosocomial infection rates have been consistently highest in large teaching hospitals and lowest in nonteaching hospitals for all services and sites of infection, suggesting that the three-level stratification effectively defines hospital categories in which patients have different levels of risk for acquiring nosocomial infections. This difference in risk undoubtedly reflects severity of underlying illness (patient mix) and the extent to which diagnostic and therapeutic procedures are performed in these hospitals.[28]

A March 1997 report of studies on nosocomial infections commissioned by the Board of Medical Device Technologies found as follows:

> Using newly developed testing procedures that simulate actual conditions in surgery, latex gloves that had passed the manufacturer's standard leak test actually allowed viruses to pass through. . . . Previous studies published in scientific and medical journals showed that more than 400 million out of 1.2 billion surgical gloves used annually in the United States lose their ability to protect against infection during a surgical procedure. These breaches could be caused by a tear, hole or small needle puncture. . . . An even greater number of gloves may be failing due to the fluid saturation of gloves. . . . The lead investigation into latex glove failure was performed by DPR Biomedical at San Diego State University. Similar results were achieved during parallel studies performed at the University of Texas Health Science Center, San Antonio and by a private testing laboratory registered by the Food and Drug Administration (FDA). . . . On average, 21 percent of the "intact" gloves tested—i.e., gloves that passed the FDA's test

for leak detection—allowed small numbers of viruses to pass through the glove. . . . Another result involved a test that pierced the gloves with a 26–gauge needle, one of the smallest used in surgeries. The FDA's test detected a leak in less than half of the pierced gloves. However, more than 90 percent of these pierced gloves allowed substantial amounts of virus to pass through within five minutes of exposure. . . . What these studies tell us is that both patient and physician need to demand better monitoring systems of their latex gloves for effective infection control.[29]

It seems clear from the foregoing that, in the last years of the twentieth century, the prevailing medical mind-set has not changed, nor has the medical scheme of ideas been altered with regard to the "dirty little secret" about hand washing and the control of nosocomial infection. These stubborn realities persist despite the fact that the continuing inattention and ignorance of medical and surgical staff is killing people at an annual rate which, as Katherine Griffin reported, is higher than that of all motor vehicle accidents and all homicides combined. It would appear that the medical guild has gone to very great lengths indeed to prevent the American public from knowing about this scandalous and quite brutal reality.

In an "Annals of Medicine" article published by the *New Yorker* magazine on September 20, 1993, Terence Monmaney reports on the discovery by J. Robin Warren, M.D., and his colleague, Barry J. Marshall, M.D., that peptic ulcers are caused by a bacterium that hides in the stomach lining. The theory

challenged widely held and seemingly unassailable notions about the cause of ulcers. No physical ailment has ever been more closely tied to psychological turbulence. "The critical factor in the development of ulcers is the frustration associated with the wish to receive love," one social scientist reported in 1983. . . . Dr. James F. Masterson states that the peptic ulcer is a "psychosomatic disorder" that typically afflicts people who are "hungering for emotional supplies that were lost in childhood or that were never sufficient to nourish the real self." . . . A highly regarded gastroenterologist declared, "It is a disease of tense, nervous persons who live a strenuous and worrisome life . . . a disease of civilization, closely linked with the tense tempo of modern life and the hurry of everyday existence." The idea of American life itself as an ulcer-causing agent runs through the medical literature. . . . According to this scenario . . . capitalist society poses all the savage threats of primitive life and yet provides none of the satisfactions.

Primed for a bloody clash that never comes, we devour our insides instead. . . . Marshall . . . presented his theory in 1983, at a gathering of infectious-disease specialists in Brussels. . . . Marshall talked about how . . . over several months he had found the bacteria in the stomach of almost every patient he saw with stomach inflammation, most patients with chronic indigestion, and almost every patient with peptic ulcer. . . . When Marshall finished speaking, an audience member stood up and gently inquired, "Dr. Marshall, what causes peptic ulcers in people who don't have the bacteria?" "If you don't have the bacteria, you don't have a peptic ulcer," Marshall said. He might as well have said he knew the secret of cold fusion. The scientists chuckled and murmured and shook their heads, a little embarrassed for a junior colleague whose debut was such a disaster. Dr. Martin Blaser, the director of the Division of Infectious Diseases at the Vanderbuilt University School of Medicine, was in the audience. Marshall's talk struck him then as "the most preposterous thing I'd ever heard . . . I thought this guy was a madman.". . . For Marshall, the trumpets of vindication sounded last February (1993), when a definitive clinical trial performed by Austrian scientists finally backed up his prediction. "Study Confirms Most Ulcers Are Caused by Bacterium, Curable by Antibiotics," *The Wall Street Journal* announced at the time. Meanwhile, field epidemiologists have been jumping into jeeps and airplanes and running off to test people all over the world for *Helicobacter* infection. They've found it everywhere. To quote a paper in *The Lancet* last fall, "*Helicobacter pylori* is arguably the commonest chronic bacterial infection in man." And, perhaps the most striking development yet, chronic *Helicobacter* infection is now recognized as a major cause of stomach cancer—the world's second most common malignancy. . . . Since the turn of the century, other medical workers . . . had glimpsed the bug, had even published microscopic pictures of stomach tissue in which these bacteria were in evidence, but they neglected to pursue it or identify it. Then, in the fifties, a supposedly definitive study of human gastrointestinal flora concluded that the stomach was microbe-free, and thus it came to be viewed as a "sterile" organ. No longer did many pathologists even bother to check the stomach for resident bacteria, and, more significant, those who found the microbe doubted their own eyes. *They did not see it because they did not believe in it.*[30] (Emphasis added)

What is perhaps most noteworthy about the reaction of the medical establishment to Marshall's discovery, and what goes furthest to explain the ten-year delay in acceptance of his valid findings, is the glaring absence of intellectual curiosity on the part of his fellow physicians. Clearly, these doctors have been trained to go "by the book," and if it isn't in the book, it should be paid no attention. This is a concrete indication of a guild whose members have been taught to ignore, and even to fear, their own first-hand clinical experience.

The Austrian researchers mentioned in Monmaney's article are now treating patients diagnosed with *H.pylori*-associated chronic duodenal ulcer with

> a combination of antibiotics and ranitidine . . . as an alternative to long-term drug-maintenance therapy or elective surgery. . . . This promises unsurpassed relief to millions of people—and considerable savings. A standard maintenance regimen of Zantac—the world's #1 prescription drug, with an estimated three billion dollars in sales last year—runs about a hundred dollars a month. Over the years, a person with a recurring ulcer might easily spend ten or fifteen thousand dollars keeping it quiet. In contrast, a twelve-day ulcer-curing course of the antibiotics amoxicillin and metronidazole, which are generic drugs, would cost about twenty dollars. All told, Marshall estimates that an ulcer can be cured outright for six hundred and fifty dollars, including the costs of visits to a physician, antibody tests, endoscopy, and drugs. . . . "Over time, within perhaps even my lifetime, we should be able to eliminate ulcer disease from the human race."[31]

Zantac was for years the expensive brand-name prescription drug of choice for the treatment of chronic stomach ulcers. As the information about Marshall's discovery spread, however, inexpensive generic antibiotics that kill *H. pylori* have entirely displaced Zantac as the appropriate ulcer medication. The manufacturers of Zantac have responded to this costly setback by producing a lower-strength version of Zantac as a nonprescription, over-the-counter product intended to combat stomach acidity.

Monmaney reports that Dr. Marshall is now studying nonulcer dyspepsia, or indigestion, which "afflicts tens of millions of Americans." He includes this trenchant and, unfortunately, apt bit of sarcasm in this part of his report: "To study the problem, Marshall has struck upon a deeply innovative medical technique: he listens to his patients and takes what they say seriously."[32] The recent experience of Barry Marshall makes evident that, as the twentieth century draws to a close, the presuppositions which continue to dominate the American medical mind remain outdated and fundamentally erroneous. There is an easy embrace of technology by physicians, and a contrary pattern of resistance by them to the acceptance of a bona fide scientific discovery on the rare occasions when this occurs in the medical field.

American Medicine in a Box Canyon

The evidence provided by the foregoing examples seems clear and convincing: "modern" medicine remains shackled to the cosmological notion of a clockwork universe and to an unacknowledged and erroneous scheme of ideas that is directly descended from the work of René Descartes. "Modern" medicine is nonetheless simultaneously continuing to *function* in a world that would be most accurately understood under a distinctly different scheme of ideas, one derived from Darwin, Einstein, nuclear physics, microbiology—a world described in terms such as organic, processive, random, pluralistic, expanding, and even infinite.

It will prove to be at least as difficult to displace and to replace the scheme of ideas that now overarches the American medical universe as it was to shift Western thought from the 1,400-year-old conceptions of Ptolemy to the revolutionary observations of Copernicus, Galileo, and Descartes. Unless this displacement occurs, however, medicine in America is unlikely to find a way out of the box canyon of the intellect that today defines the limits of its forward progress as a science.

The scheme of ideas that one may divine from a study of contemporary medical education and practice is laced with erroneous assumptions and wrongheaded notions, but because this scheme of ideas is unacknowleged by the medical profession, and is therefore never made explicit, medicine has not found it possible to evaluate or to criticize—and thereby improve—the ideas that form its foundations. For as long as this condition persists, medical inquiry in the United States will continue to find itself boxed in. And, for as long as this condition persists, organized medicine in America will continue to build its technological capacities, and will continue unfailingly to mistake technological inventions for real medical science.

Here is the true source of the major crisis in American medicine, and the crisis is today at the critical stage.

The Important Difference
Between Science and Technology

Lewis Thomas, M.D., former chairman of pathology and dean at Yale Medical School, and former president of Memorial Sloan Kettering Cancer Center in New York City, a man who calls himself a "biology watcher," has provided his own assessment of the technological developments in medicine which have been so impressive for the society during the past fifty years.[33] He has separated medical technology into three distinct and quite different levels: the first is "nontechnology" which he defines as the attentive and even reverential caring that physicians sometimes extend to their patients, what Thomas terms "supportive therapy"—not subject to measurement in terms of its impact on the outcomes of an illness; the next level is "halfway technology" which Thomas describes as medical or surgical interventions intended to ameliorate the effects of a disease that we cannot cure, and to forestall death from that disease. Organ transplants would represent the most dramatic example of "halfway technology." Thomas declares this level of medical technology to be at once "highly sophisticated and profoundly primitive." It is also the aspect of contemporary medical technology that propels expenditures by society, as well as income for physicians, to stratospheric heights. The final level he calls "the real high technology of medicine . . . [that] comes as the result of a genuine understanding of disease mechanisms." Thomas points out that the breakthrough technologies at this level —vaccines, for example—have proven to be relatively inexpensive, and relatively easy to deliver to patients. He provides a particularly trenchant comparison of levels two and three—"half technology" and "high technology":

> The halfway technology that was evolving for poliomyelitis in the early 1950s, just before the emergence of the basic research that made the vaccine possible, provides another illustration of the point. Do you remember Sister Kenny, and the cost of those institutions for rehabilitation, with all those ceremonially applied hot fomentations, and the debates about whether the affected limbs should be totally immobilized or kept in passive motion as frequently as possible, and the masses of statistically tormented data mobilized to support one view or the other? It is the cost of that kind of technology, and its relative effectiveness, that must be com-

pared with the cost and effectiveness of the [polio] vaccine. . . . It is when physicians are bogged down by their incomplete technologies, by the innumerable things they are obliged to do in medicine when they lack a clear understanding of disease mechanisms, that the deficiencies of the health-care system are most conspicuous.[33]

In the four sentences quoted above, Thomas uses the recent history of American approaches to the treatment of poliomyelitis to point out the pivotal difference between a technological invention and a scientific breakthrough; and to emphasize the point that cost comparisons between today's open-ended varieties of medical technology, on one hand, and real scientific breakthroughs such as the polio vaccine, on the other hand, merit careful analysis and serious consideration by everyone who bears any part of the gigantic financial burden now imposed on American society by the medical-care system. Lewis Thomas reminds us that thanks to the work of Albert Sabin, among others, medicine gained the ability to prevent a ravaging disease in the entire human population at a cost of pennies per individual, a disease which, absent the vaccine, would otherwise have by this time cost billions to treat, with no end in sight to the human suffering or to the steady escalation of expenditures on treatment.

When Thomas's three levels of medical technology are looked at from the viewpoint that American medicine is proceeding on the basis of an erroneous cosmology and an erroneous epistemology, a clearer light may be shed on his analysis by slightly altering his three labels. Instead of nontechnology, the first category can be termed "nonscience," at least "nonbiologic science"; the second category merits the same label, "nonscience," and can accurately be termed "technology"; and the third category, which Thomas has called "high technology," is the only one which would merit the title "science," or "biologic science," or, within this context, "medical science."

It is particularly noteworthy that during the last decade of the twentieth century, American physicians have convinced themselves, and most of the nonmedical public, that improvements in technology represent the highest state of the art and science of medicine. These are the technological advances which fall under Dr. Thomas's second category of "halfway technology," the ones which are being marketed to the American public as the highest-level achievements of medical science. Furthermore, it is important to note that all

of the examples which Lewis Thomas provides in his category of "high technology" have resulted from the work of biologists, pathologists, and chemists
—people whose experience in their specific field of inquiry has led them to a
cosmology and an epistemology which are shot through with organic, processive, random, pluralistic and relational characteristics. Their scheme of ideas
reflects a radical difference from the notions of a mechanistic or clockwork
universe, and this fact is of central importance to their scientific imaginations
and to the beneficial insights and discoveries their imaginings have produced
in the field of medicine. Only the breakthroughs in Thomas's third category
of "high technology" flow from a medical scheme of ideas which gives full and
conscious sway to organism and to process as the most pervasive and persuasive facts about the nature of reality. The word "science" should be substituted
for the term "high technology" in order to make crystal clear the significant
distinction between diseases that medicine has discovered a means to prevent
or to cure, and the many prevalent diseases which modern medicine "cannot
cure: cardiovascular disease, most cancers, arthritis, multiple sclerosis, stroke,
advanced cirrhosis, and the common cold."[34]

It would not be unreasonable to conclude from the foregoing that in
order to achieve rapid and continuous future discoveries in medical science,
as contrasted with additions to medical technology, there will have to be a
thoroughgoing reconstruction of the scheme of ideas on which American
medicine is basing itself today.

Abraham Flexner: An Outstanding Coup

Before considering what the outlines of a reconstructed medical care system
would look like on the threshold of the twenty-first century, a review is in
order of the massive reconstruction of medical education—and, simultaneously, of guild rubrics and power—which was undertaken in 1910 by the
AMA's Council on Education in conjunction with Abraham Flexner.

As the twentieth century got underway, there was no doubt in Abraham
Flexner's mind that thoroughgoing reconstruction of medical education
would be essential if improvement in medical care was to occur in the United
States. Flexner recommended that the proposed reconstruction be accomplished through licensure and accreditation powers delegated to medical

boards in each state, and through a radical reconfiguration of medical education. The medical guild, represented by the AMA's Council on Education, wholeheartedly supported Flexner's approach. *The Flexner Report*, published in 1910, promulgated a new "cosmology" and scheme of ideas for medicine in the United States, and as Flexner's proposals were implemented, the American medical cosmos assumed many new and distinct characteristics. The American medical guild seized the opportunity provided by the *Flexner Report* as their occasion to reconstruct the medical cosmos in a manner which would:

(a) overcome the perception that medicine in the United States was inferior to European medicine;

(b) reduce competition for the medical care dollar by using state licensure to drastically cut the number of practicing physicians; and

(c) provide a means of coping with the post-Darwinian explosion of knowledge through the expansion of medical "specialization."

The medical guild therefore strongly supported the widespread implementation of Flexner's report during the second decade of the century, the roaring twenties, and the thirties, in what amounted to medicine's version of a Copernican Revolution. For most of the first three centuries in America, the general physician had occupied the center of the medical universe, and the bedroom of his ill or injured patient had most often been the locus for the provision of his most critical services. The reordering of the medical universe, which flowed from Flexner's report, displaced the general physician from his central role and placed the hospital—the workshop of the free-baron "specialists"—at the center of the medical cosmos, with every other entity or resource being defined with reference to this new center of gravitational power.

The impact of the *Flexner Report* on "specialization" has had a number of devastating effects on medicine in America. The explosion of medical specialties effectively drove the generalist physicians from the universities as too ill-informed to be worthy of participation. Medicine has yet to address, much less overcome, the resulting bifurcation of the community of inquiry in medical science. Channels of inquiry, of learning and of teaching, no matter how deep they may be, require the kind of integration with the entire *corpus* of inquiry, across all special fields of knowledge, which only the generalist mind-set is likely to bring about.

Under this "new" scheme of ideas, with the hospital installed at the center of the medical universe, and with the various departments of the university medical school as its orbiting heavenly partners, the arrangement of the bodies in orbit became hierarchical—emphasizing the distinction of one category of "specialist" physician from another, and deemphasizing the relationships between and among them. The most important "specialists" enjoyed the inner orbit about the hospital center, and vice versa.

State medical boards were stacked with "specialists" and armed with direct power to license physicians and to accredit medical schools, which had to be within a university, or formally affiliated with an established, reputable university.

Generalist physicians, who had been in control of American medicine from the seventeenth century until 1910, were now viewed as second- or third-class players, and as a source of some embarrassment to the profession. They found themselves pushed to the extreme edges of this new medical cosmos. Like the earth itself after Galileo, the generalist was transformed into "a third-rate planet of a second-rate star." To this day, and despite residencies in "Family Practice" having been established in many university medical schools as a new field of "specialization," general physicians have not yet overcome their re-situation on the outermost edges of the new medical cosmos; and "organized" medicine in the United States has virtually no comprehension of the great harm it has thereby done to itself.

The generalists had traditionally considered surgery as one relatively minor aspect of a general practice. These doctors now discovered that, in the world where university-related medical schools and their "workshops"—the hospitals—occupied the central position, surgery rapidly became the predominant "specialty." As the center of the new American medical cosmos, the hospital assumed the central role in the rapidly expanding system of "specialized" medical services. The decision to separate the person from their normal environment by admitting them to a hospital mirrors the "specialist" mind-set, which tends to separate the disease from the person, and the critical event from the enduring process. The most extreme examples of this bifurcation of human persons from the maladies that afflict them have been provided by the most radical of the surgical "specialists"; however, all surgeons, to some degree, participate in this fundamentally fallacious view.

The American breakthroughs in anesthesia—initially chloroform and ether—made possible the swift rise of the surgeon. Had surgery remained the painful, often horrible procedure it had been before anesthesia, patient volume would have remained low, and surgery would have remained a relatively rare practice. With the advent of "painless" surgery, however, surgeons rapidly became the principal source of revenue for the hospitals and their affiliated medical schools.

The surgeon's transition from the barbershops of the old world, when in the eyes of "doctors of medicine" they did not merit the title of physician, to the attainment of the highest position on the medical totem in the New World, was now complete. For their unwillingness or inability to qualify as "specialists," the generalists were virtually banished from the university medical schools.

The massive insecurity complex American physicians had traditionally harbored vis-à-vis European medicine could now be effectively overcome as the direct result of university-based production of "specialties" and of "specialists" on the overwhelming scale that Europe has, in general, come to expect of America. A larger and larger proportion of licensed physicians in the United States would become "diplomate specialists"; i.e., in addition to their degree as a medical doctor, these physicians would hold an additional diploma issued by one of the "specialty" academies, such as the American Academy of Radiologists, or the American College of Surgeons—or any of the other eighty-odd academies in business today. In the view of the free barons of medicine on this continent, European medicine would thereby be surpassed, and its criticisms silenced. The geometric increase in "specialization" during the past century, which has been unique to the United States, could be construed in part as being a defense against the longstanding denigration of American physicians by the medical guild of Europe. The newly reconstructed medical guild in the United States could only view this turn of events as an outstanding coup for American "specialism."

More than any other single factor, however, the channeling of medical inquiry into "specialties," coupled with the presupposition that the distinctions between one field of medicine and another are far more significant than any relationships across different fields of inquiry, has condemned "modern" medicine to its current pathway, a route that has steadfastly led the American medical "community of inquiry" directly to the ideological box canyon in which it is now entrapped.

The timing of this crossroads opportunity for American medicine to rev-
olutionize itself was truly extraordinary. The watershed of information about
the human organism following the publication of Darwin's *Origin of Species* in
1859 made the inadequacy of the then-existing medical schools in the
United States even more vivid. Darwinism produced an outflow of new information about the human species, and as it came forth, new "specialty" fields
were rapidly identified and labeled. The large pool of American doctors
could be re-sorted, the more academically inclined being selected for training
in a "specialized" field, with one consequence being a reduction of the competitive pressures felt by the doctors who remained in general practice. "Specialization" seemed an entirely logical response to the flood of new information after 1859, and to the consequent inability of any one physician to
master all of the available knowledge.

The *Flexner Report* has been seen as the turning point at which American
medicine: "became a scientifically based discipline."[35] New and reconstructed
medical schools—tied to major universities—with "generalism" banished
from their reordered world, established specialization as the cornerstone of a
"scientific" approach to the practice of medicine. This single decision proved
to be the principal contributing cause of the mistaking of technological
invention for scientific breakthrough, and of the replacement of a public
health focus by a virtually exclusive concern with the provision of medical
services to individuals. As a corollary of this new scheme, the radical shift in
focus and concern by "specialist" physicians has also fostered the unprecedented and pervasive growth of commercialism in American medicine, and
the virtual disappearance of previously perceived limits to the manifestation
of greed on the part of physicians. This single decision to banish and denigrate generalism can thus be seen as the wellspring of the patterns of cyni-
cism and intellectual dishonesty which have come to characterize too many
dimensions of contemporary medical practice. The rod of correction that the
generalist cast of mind could provide within the community of inquiry has
been lost.

Continuously nourished from the fountainhead of Darwinism, "specialties" have been flooding in, followed quickly by subspecialties, and subsub-
specialties. Generalists with their integrated minds got the message from the
now-dominant "specialists" of the medical guild's academies that they need
not apply. The new medical cosmos would forcefully prefer those physicians

who understood their role and purpose as being narrowly focused curers of individual episodes of disease; and, above all else, as victors over death.

A few brief selections from the 1910 *Flexner Report* will provide a more vivid picture of the condition of American medicine, and of medical education in the United States, as this revolution got underway less than nine decades ago:

> [T]he creation of [the proprietary] type [of medical school] was the fertile source of unforeseen harm to medical education and to medical practice. . . . Between 1810 and 1840, twenty-six new medical schools sprang up; between 1840 and 1876, forty-seven more; and the number actually surviving in 1876 has been since then much more than doubled. . . . [T]he United States and Canada have in little more than a century produced four hundred and fifty-seven medical schools. One hundred and fifty-five survive today [i.e., 1910].[36]

> The one hundred and fifty-five medical schools . . . fall readily into three divisions: the first includes those that require two or more years of college work for entrance; the second, those that demand actual graduation from a four-year high school or oscillate about its supposed "equivalent"; the third, those that ask little or nothing more than the rudiments or the recollection of a common school education.[37]

> We have indeed in America medical practitioners not inferior to the best elsewhere; but there is probably no other country in the world in which there is so great a distance and so fatal a difference between the best, the average, and the worst.[38]

> As a matter of fact, many of the schools mentioned in the course of this recital are probably without redeeming features of any kind. . . . The teaching is an uninstructive rehearsal of textbook or quiz-compend. . . . Third- and fourth-year men are frequently huddled together in the same classes. . . . So much for the worst.[39]

> The necessity of a reconstruction that will at once reduce the number and improve the output of medical schools may now be taken as demonstrated. . . . The principles upon which reconstruction would proceed have been established in the course of this report: (1) a medical school is properly a university department; it is most favorably located in a large city, where the problem of procuring clinical material (i.e., patients), at once abundant and

various, practically solves itself. Hence those universities that have been located in cities can most advantageously develop medical schools. . . . The schools of Albany, Buffalo, Brooklyn, Washington, would, on this plan, disappear,—certainly until academic institutions of proper caliber had been developed. . . . [B]etter state laws are needed in order to exterminate the worst schools; merger or liquidation must bring together many of those that still survive. . . . In the north central tier . . . population increased 239,685 the last year: 160 doctors would care for the increase.[40]

It is significant to note that, in 1910, Flexner believed that the proper ratio of physicians to population should be 67 doctors per 100,000 people. The current ratio in the United States is over 240 per 100,000, and based upon the rate at which physicians are being produced in this country, the ratio is projected to be 290 per 100,000 within the next seven years. That would be over four times what Flexner considered reasonable and proper in 1910.

Reduction of our 155 medical schools to 31 would deprive of a medical school no section that is now capable of maintaining one. It would threaten no scarcity of physicians until the country's development actually required more than 3500 physicians annually, that is to say, for a generation or two, at least . . . and every institution arranged for can be expected to make some useful contribution to knowledge and progress. The postgraduate school as developed in the United States may be characterized as a "compensatory adjustment." It is an effort to mend a machine that was predestined to break down. Inevitably, the more conscientious and intelligent men trained in most of the medical schools herein described must become aware of their unfitness for the responsibilities of medical practice; the postgraduate school was established to do what the medical school had failed to accomplish. . . . The postgraduate school was thus originally an undergraduate repair shop. . . . Postgraduate, like other schools, vary in character. . . . The Brooklyn Postgraduate School, for instance, entertains less than half a dozen students on the average at a time, in a wretched hospital, really a death-trap, heavily laden with debt, and without laboratory equipment enough to make an ordinary clinical examination.[41]

The state boards are the instruments through which the reconstruction of medical education will be largely effected. To them the graduate in medicine applies for the license to practice. Their power can be both indirectly and directly exerted. . . . No institution can long survive the day upon which it is . . . publicly branded as feeble, unfit, or disreputable. . . . [T]he arm of the state boards should for the present go beyond the rejection of individuals to the actual closing up of notoriously incompetent institutions. The law that protects the public against the unfit doctor should in fairness protect the student against the unfit school. . . . [S]o long as any group of physicians may in most states incorporate a medical school under general laws that offer no safeguard at all, and licensure examinations are not yet deliberately constructed to frustrate their activity, summary protective power against mercenary and incompetent faculties must be lodged somewhere. The boards therefore touch at three points the problems with which this report has dealt: for they deal: (1) with the preliminary educational requirement, (2) with the facilities of medical schools, (3) with examinations for licensure. . . . Of such overwhelming importance . . . is the character of the license examination that, if thorough practical examinations were instituted, all the other perplexing details . . . would become relatively immaterial. How far we are now from this ideal realized in other countries, hardly aspired to in America, a few facts make plain. In 1906, the worst of the Chicago schools—a school with no entrance requirement, no laboratory teaching, no hospital connections—made before state boards the best record attained by any Chicago school in that year. . . . To do their duty fully, the state boards require to be properly constituted, organized, and equipped. At present, none of them fulfills all these conditions.[42]

In any analysis of the status of medicine and of medical education in contemporary America, it would be well to recognize and remember that these words of Abraham Flexner's were written just eighty-eight years ago.

The new medical establishment did not, however, take all of Flexner's ideas to heart, making no provision in its reordered medical cosmos for the primacy that Flexner assigned to the medical care of the general population—the public interest:

The overwhelming importance of preventive medicine, sanitation, and public health indicates that in modern life the medical profession is an organ differentiated by society for its own highest purposes, not a business to be exploited by individuals according to their own fancy. There would be no more vigorous campaigns led by enlightened practitioners against tuberculosis, malaria, and diphtheria, if the commercial point of view were tolerable in practice. And if not in practice, then not in education. The theory of state regulation covers that point. In the act of granting the right to confer degrees, the state vouches for them; through protective boards it still further seeks to safeguard the people. The public interest is then paramount, and when public interest, professional ideals, and sound educational procedure concur in the recommendation of the same policy, the time is surely ripe for decisive action.[43]

Medicine's Comfort with the "Commercial Viewpoint"

As the twentieth century comes to a close, the evidence is overwhelming that the members of the American guild most assuredly find the "commercial point of view . . . tolerable in practice"; indeed it is now the cornerstone of building a medical practice. What Abraham Flexner would have to say about the fact that about forty million Americans lack regular access to routine medical care, despite a massive physician oversupply, would amount to an earful that the contemporary medical guild membership would surely not want to hear. But what Flexner did not understand is that specialization emphasizes technical knowledge and mechanical skill: hand-eye coordination, for example; and that "specialism" concentrates attention on the categorical medical event, while overlooking the continuous and processive aspects of disease. The scheme of ideas overarching the dramatic movement into specialization is fundamentally mechanistic and dualistic, and not organic. Healing is thus viewed as a technical and industrial process best accomplished in a medical workshop, a factory. The primary object of medical inquiry thereby becomes the part, the unit, the system, or the aspect. The pivotal contribution of "specialism" has been to break things down, to focus on organs—the heart, the kidney, the liver—as central in importance.

The continuation of "life" is recognized as the goal above all others: however, "life" is defined for the medical specialist in technical terms, as victory over death. Can a brain wave be detected? Then, there is life, and death has been defied. For contemporary American medicine, "life" has been redefined so as to accommodate the worldview of the super-surgeons; and "death" has been redefined by the "specialist" as a technical defeat for the attending physician. Irrespective of the age or condition of a patient, death is not to be viewed by the physician as the completion of a natural process undergone by a human being.

The redefinition of human death as a technical defeat *for the medical specialist* is a logical consequence of the erroneous epistemology of the contemporary "specialist" physician. Paul Starr, a Harvard sociologist and the author of an insightful book entitled *The Social Transformation of American Medicine*, offers this comment:

> A French physician (Jean Hamburger) calls it "therapeutic relentlessness." In its commitment to the preservation of life, medical care ironically has come to symbolize a prototypically modern form of torture, combining benevolence, indifference, and technical wizardry. Rather than engendering trust, technological medicine often raises anxieties about the ability of individuals to make choices for themselves.[44]

Ask super-surgeons how they would like to die, and it becomes clear that the ending they wish for themselves is always quite different than being tubed and wired up in the intensive care unit of a hospital, with their fate in the hands of a death defier. Some years ago, while talking with several super-surgeons in a faculty lounge at Pennsylvania Hospital, the news came that a friend we had all been with the day before had died of a major cerebral aneurysm during his sleep. He was eighty five, and enjoyed an international reputation as an immunologist. It was devastating news for me, however my physician companions were right on the verge of being joyous, because of the *way* in which our friend had died. "What a way to go," one said. Their feeling was that he had been at full throttle the day before in meetings, and then he was gone in his sleep, without an ache or a pain, and without being in an ER or a hospital bed. "What a lucky SOB," another said. These were the sentiments of his fellow physicians, who had great affection for the man.

If you ask physicians how they would like to die, you'll learn that it would NOT be as the result of a technical defeat on the part of a medical colleague. The general preference is to experience death as, pure and simple, a natural event, preferably undergone in a normal environment, in contact and communication with loved ones, with ample opportunity to say goodbye. Or, suddenly, like our friend.

It should come as no surprise, however, that the medical "specialist" in the

United States has tended to take a sharp intellectual turn away from any need to demonstrate concern for individual patients in a manner that could be construed as "reverent" in the interpersonal sphere. These specific dimensions of medicine are being consciously left to general practitioners, who are categorized by contemporary graduate medical educators as scoring high on the "socio-emotional" index. That is to say, although the generalists may not be the brightest of the graduate medical students (otherwise, why would they become generalists?), they do tend to care about their patients as human persons.

Scheme B, above, shoving the generalist physician to the edges of the medical cosmos, is the theory that propelled "specialist" physicians to the forefront of power and influence, derived from the seventeenth century thinking of René Descartes: a fundamentally mechanistic, dualistic theory; a clockwork universe giving primacy to the mechanical tasks of removing and replacing parts.

This splitting up of the aspects of "human being" which can only be fully comprehended in the fullness of their connectedness and coherence is the root cause of the crisis in thinking which exists today in the field of medicine. Although himself a student of medicine, Descartes may be judged as perhaps the outstanding villain in steering Western thinking down this particular blind alley.

Supported by its Cartesian scheme of ideas, medical inquiry in the United States has adopted as its *central position,* its central focus, the "specialized" study and treatment of the human body perceived as an object, as a thing, as a machine. Mechanism lies at the very heart of contemporary American medical epistemology. It is no wonder, therefore, that the surgeon—the master mechanic—has come to occupy the highest rank in the professional hierarchy of American medicine for most of this century. And it is no wonder that the biochemist and the human physiologist—for whom the human body is a wondrously complex, fully autonomous and still mysterious chemical factory—have been viewed with indifference by physicians in practice, as people engaged in research activities rarely having relevance to the daily task of the saving of human lives, and therefore as people basically divorced from the profession of the practicing "specialist" physician.

In the age of specialists, and under the unacknowledged influence of a mechanistic theory, American medicine has lost sight of, and has gone without, a valid "central position." To quote my teacher, Robert C. Pollock, from his essay on Emerson:

Emerson knew that if men shunned what was most valuable in their experience, it was because they had accepted the fiction of a split universe. ... In other words, Emerson was determined to cast out the devils of the mechanistic outlook which had alienated men from their own deeper experiences.[45]

In medicine, the *central position* ought to be a full-blown, true, untrammeled and *generalist* focus upon *scientific* inquiry, openly dedicated to serving the best interests of the patient—all things being considered, and nothing being omitted. Instead, American medicine is the captive of its decision, reflecting medical guild perceptions of the dictates of the *Flexner Report*, to glorify the all-knowing medical "specialist," and to denigrate the generalist. Curiosity and receptiveness to new insight ought to be central, but as we have seen, they most assuredly are not.

From the Barbershop to "Top Gun" Status

The general physician as caregiver is, and has always been, a conserver, widely recognized within the culture for dealing with ill or injured persons in a reverent manner. Physician caregivers have always been true conservatives.

Surgical "specialists," on the other hand, clearly are the most dedicated death defiers in medicine. In contrast with physicians who view their role as caregivers, the death-defying surgeon is a true radical. Virtually anything goes. The prevailing attitude is: "If we can do it, it ought to be done." The primary purpose is to achieve a victory over death one more time. In an explicitly radical subversion of the Hippocratic Oath that each physician is sworn to uphold at graduation from medical school, the surgical specialists have decreed that causing harm to 50 percent of your patients is okay. That is, if the projected "success rate" (i.e., the five-year survival rate) for a given surgical procedure is fifty-fifty, that constitutes a valid basis for proceeding to operate. From the surgeon's standpoint, after all, that's a batting average of .500, which isn't half bad, depending upon your vantage point. Surgeons have most assuredly exhibited some bizarre viewpoints about the care of patients, and the harm caused to them. Take for example surgeon John Hall, M.D., the Chief of Medical Staff of the British Expeditionary Army in the

Crimean War, who wrote in his 1854 letter of instructions to his medical officers: "The smart use of the knife is a powerful stimulant and it is much better to hear a man bawl lustily than to see him sink silently into the grave." The letter was written only a few years after surgeons had begun using anesthesia, and Dr. Hall clearly did not consider this discovery a boon to his surgical practice.

What Hippocrates had in mind was causing *no* harm, *none at all* to the patient. The consistent behavior of the American radicals in greens, however, reveals the fact that their medical "science" has transported them beyond the pale of concern with a patient's feelings or preferences; or of concern with personalities, with families, or even with the most concrete manifestations of pain and suffering; and has brought them to the point of *expecting* risk, as their patients must learn to do. Victory over death—there's the thing that matters most to a surgeon. Await sickness, await disease or disability—and then move in to "save" individual lives.

Not the most caring people go into surgery. Technical excellence is the key requirement. It takes a certain arrogance to cut open the body of another human being. Surgeons prefer to view this aspect of their demeanor as indicative of their professional confidence. Prior to the discovery of anesthesia, surgery meant intense pain and suffering for the surgical patients. In the late nineteenth century and the early part of this century, surgeries were often witnessed by surgical residents and other medical students. This meant that excruciating human pain and suffering were being witnessed as well. These theatric performances by renowned surgeons set the mold for proper behavior during the performance of surgical procedures without benefit of anaesthesia: the surgeon must consistently demonstrate to all present that he is completely untouched by and impervious to human suffering, and can remain indifferent to the agonies his patient is experiencing under his knife. The patient must be viewed as a machine to be repaired, or as a slab of meat to be cut upon. The pain and suffering was not always a bloody affair. Bone setting was poorly understood by physicians, with the result that surgeons in this period at places like Harvard, Johns Hopkins, and Pennsylvania would attempt to reset a hipbone which had been dislocated from its socket six months previously. It always proved impossible, of course, but many an aspiring surgical resident passed out at witnessing the screams of the patient being victimized by such a procedure.

To a "top gun" surgeon, bedside manner has become irrelevant from a professional point of view. Repair or replacement of the part is what counts. Fixing the machine is what counts. Victory over death is what counts. The principal goal is to avoid the medical defeat, which the death of the patient would represent. Because of the deeply ingrained arrogance that has become characteristic of their profession, most surgical "specialists" have simply lost sight of the affective dimension, and of its importance for human healing and wellness. The most frequent descriptives whispered about surgeons by those on the inside are: insensitive, dictatorial, arrogant, and God complex. In fact, there are otherwise reputable surgeons who are openly quite proud of the fact that they personally have earned and indeed merit these descriptives.

And who else in the spectrum of medical specialties achieves the most dramatic victories over death? Who can replace one essential part with a different one, without ever recognizing that each attempted organ transplant, and each coronary artery bypass operation is rooted in a public health failure of some kind? Rather, these arrogant radicals spend their time hoping, praying, and working hard to secure unto themselves a more abundant harvest of spare parts to draw upon.

It is worthy of note that the surgical death-defiers whose business is transplant surgery are prepared to more readily accept the finality of "brain death" whenever the patient is the potential donor of organs needed for transplantation. The American "top guns" understand fully that a donor organ must be "sufficiently intact" for transplant, meaning that it must be harvested early. Going to extremes to defy death for a potential organ donor lacks the appeal which would otherwise be present. This is a clear, if rather grisly, example of what John Wennberg, M.D. has termed "practice style," and it is a culturally driven phenomenon.

In Japan, by way of contrast, organ transplants are extremely rare. Shinto belief holds that death does not occur until *all organs have expired,* which is to say until all organs have become useless for transplanting into another person. This ancient Shinto belief is not likely to change easily, therefore, despite the efforts of a cadre of high-tech surgeons, Japanese culture will undoubtedly be pursuing a very different path with regard to organ transplants than the one that American culture has already enthusiastically embarked upon.

In a book entitled *The Unkindest Cut: Life in the Backrooms of Medicine,* published in 1977, Marcia Millman wrote:

The manner in which coronary bypass surgery developed in the United States reflects the laissez-faire attitudes and structures that characterize American medicine. Two facts are central in this matter. First, there are no restrictions on how experimental surgical procedures can be used in American medicine. Second, . . . it is generally the case that surgeons loyally support one another in resisting any regulation or restriction on surgical practice.[46]

In May 1977 Dr. Christian Barnard, the surgeon who performed the world's first heart transplant, made the following statements about bypass surgery to a meeting of his medical colleagues, responding to a question about why physicians seemed reluctant to express any criticism of the operation:

There is no other operation in the treatment of heart disease more misused than coronary artery surgery. You can earn a lot as a coronary artery surgeon. Second, it's a very easy operation technically, and in many cases the patients do well even if you don't do anything. I would predict that if coronary artery surgery were made illegal in the world today, half the heart surgeons would be out of business and would have to beg for their money, because they exist on this type of surgery.[47]

Herbert Bauer, M.D., a specialist in public health and population medicine, appeared before a Blue Ribbon panel on open-heart surgery and stated that, after all the miraculous things that have been done in cardiovascular surgery in the United States, it can be said with full confidence that there has not been one instance in which a person has been enabled to prevent cardiovascular disease as a result of medical interventions by cardiovascular surgeons.

In the United States, we have billions to spend for bypass surgeries and heart transplants, but not even one percent of that money to invest in the prevention of cardiovascular disease. Ask nutritional therapists or exercise physiologists the question: Can you prevent cardiovascular disease? and they answer promptly in the affirmative. Cardiovascular surgeons, on the other hand, respond to the same question by posing two principal questions of their own: How can I derive an income from doing that? and: How could I possibly claim the credit for doing that? The predominant interests of the preeminent "specialists" in American medicine clearly lie with cash income and with psychological payoffs. These surgeons may be considered the "top guns" of medicine, but they surely are not in possession of the "right stuff."

It cannot make their nonsurgical colleagues proud to recognize that these twin interests—cash income and psychological payoffs—suffice to define for us the *central position* of the "specialist" physicians who continue to occupy the very pinnacle of the professional hierarchy in American medicine today.

Nonetheless, these celebrated fighter pilots of medicine are now on top, financially and otherwise. In spite of recently issued federal guidelines and standards recommending that patients be provided with full information about all of the treatment options available to them, expressed in the language they normally use and including the option of no treatment whenever it is appropriate, the realities of the medical marketplace today continue to reflect the well-worn adage which physicians who are not surgeons have used among themselves: if you go to a surgeon, you'll get a surgical solution. The decision to operate is very rarely, if ever, a consumer decision. As things stand today, it is a rare surgeon who will take the time to provide the patient with the opportunity to express a preference among alternatives, with at least one of their options being a nonsurgical choice. It remains a difficult challenge for the surgeon to step back from their own treatment preference, and to give the patient the information and the space to express their own preference. It also remains true that no other actor in fee-based medicine has an economic incentive to say no to a decision to operate. The actual result is that there is plenty of unnecessary cutting being done, resulting in more morbidity and mortality, and in a general *decrease* in the health status of the population.

However, a very different, and contrary, result has been widely broadcast and effectively marketed in the land. Combining the erroneous cosmology of a clockwork universe and an erroneous epistemology shot through with Cartesian mechanism, these physicians have convinced themselves that the highest medical art is one in which mechanical skills predominate. These surgeons see themselves as the master mechanics of the human body—immobilizing the machine in their sterile workshops, the hospitals—repairing, servicing, replacing parts on a standardized basis. The shortage of parts is regularly deplored. There is a drive underway to include on all drivers licenses permission to harvest organs from accident victims. This mind-set could conceivably lead transplant surgeons to advocate the repeal of seat-belt laws.

Simplemindedness in the Media

What makes matters much worse is the fact that the "top guns" of the medical profession have completely hoodwinked the congenitally gullible fourth estate. Journalists have been taken in by the life-or-death escapades of medicine's fighter pilots, and they have been co-opted into persuading the American public that the surgical wizardry of these death-defying physicians, in all of its technical, mechanical, and industrial proficiency, has led to high health standards for the American population, and holds some promise for the future health status of the people of the United States. These super-specialist surgeons are being presented as the reason that this country "enjoys the best health care in the world."

By this point, it ought to be evident to the reader that what we face in these haughty assertions is a set of damnable lies. The question that should be posed is: Where's the medical science? The facts are quite distinctly otherwise than the journalists have gotten them. Public-health measures—the control of infectious diseases, improved sanitation, clean water, breakthroughs in pharmacology—these are the biomedical factors that have accounted for improvements in health status for Americans. In all of these respects, death is defied in a much less immediate and less visible manner. Unlike transplant surgery, this is not the stuff of headlines, but it is the true heart of medicine.

The fourth estate never fails to demonstrate its general dullness and lack of insight in reporting on "leading-edge" surgical exploits. Reporters consistently celebrate the medical mechanics as heroes: the surgeon and assistant surgeon are pictured on the front page whenever a local heart transplant has been done, and the patient has come through it alive. However, the more subtle scientific minds that account for the real breakthroughs, the hematologists and immunologists who conquer the truly difficult problem of rejection, are never mentioned, let alone seen. These true medical scientists, fighting against the complex rejection processes of the human body, are never mentioned in media accounts of heroic surgical transplantation feats; and they are lucky if their annual income reaches 10 percent of the income the average cardiovascular surgeon enjoys.

The working press is not likely to ever report that the fourth leading cause of death in the United States, right behind heart disease, cancer, and stroke, is infections acquired after admission to a hospital. These hospital-acquired infections result mainly from the failure of medical staff to follow the prescribed aseptic procedures, including a failure by physicians and nurses to wash their hands and wear sterile gloves when examining or treating patients. As noted above, these infections kill more Americans each year than the number who lose their lives to homicides and auto accidents combined. Nonetheless, there will be no headlines.

For journalism, the standing rule is: headline the death-defier, by all means. That constitutes news. Death that is not defied, perhaps as the result of hospital-acquired infection, is relatively boring. The hypocrisy and the absence of insight on the part of journalists and their editors should come as no surprise. It is nothing other than what hard experience will teach one to expect from contemporary reporters and commentators. Casey Stengel told a story that perfectly illustrates the expectation this culture should have when it comes to the intellectual abilities of the working press. Stengel told of being grabbed by a reporter right after Don Larsen had completed the only perfect game ever pitched in a world series, and one of only fourteen perfect games ever pitched up to that moment. The reporter's question of the manager was: Is this the best game Larsen has pitched?

The gullibility and dullness of the fourth estate have combined with the arrogance of "top gun" surgeons to put surgery at the top of the medical totem in the United States, while the true medical scientists involved in these procedures are simply ignored. The fighter pilots of medicine provide perfect grist for the mindless mills of the fourth estate, with the result that most Americans have been terribly misled; and the facts about a major system of services upon which the society depends have been twisted and distorted so severely that straightening them out in the popular mind may not be possible.

The media and the general public have not been alone: every other subdivision of medicine has given its recognition to the dramatic victories over death achieved by surgeons engaged in transplanting organs. Many of their medical colleagues have been cheering from the sidelines as the super-surgeons have carved themselves into place at the top of the medical totem pole. The principal skills that these surgeons bring to the table are manual dexterity, a knowledge of anatomy, and a good memory. The fame and glory these skills have obtained for them has multiplied the financial returns to medicine's showhorses, which has generated a countervailing downward pressure on the economic status of the system's workhorses, especially those "socio-emotional" generalist physicians who see twenty-five or thirty patients a day in the office.

In a not unfamiliar pattern for American culture, the rich surgeons are getting richer, which influences many of the "brighter" medical students to choose the surgical specialties, and which has been causing dedicated family physicians to advise their children against following in their footsteps. The inevitable, albeit entirely irrational, result is that the oversupply of surgeons is increasing rapidly, in direct proportion to the increase in the relative shortage of primary care physicians.

Radical Variation in Medical Practice

While the American Medical Association has reported the median annual physician income for 1995 as being $150,000, there are cardiovascular surgeons committed exclusively to coronary artery bypass surgery with annual incomes in 1995 as high as four million dollars. There are ophthalmologists, specializing in cataract surgery, who easily bring in seven figure incomes. Surely, the technical skills of these surgeons have value, and the society wants and needs the valuable medical services they can provide. The major problem stems from the structure of the medical cosmos that has spawned these physicians; from the scheme of ideas the physicians have derived from this cosmos; and from the erroneous epistemology which alone can explain the frightening phenomenon of extreme variation in what Dr. John Wennberg of Dartmouth has termed "practice style":

> I have observed that in Maine, by the time women reach seventy years of age in one hospital market, the likelihood they have undergone a hysterectomy is 20 percent; while in another market it is 70 percent. In Iowa, the chances that male residents who reach age eighty-five have undergone prostatectomy range from a low of 15 percent to a high of more than 60 percent in different hospital markets. In Vermont, the probability that resident children will undergo a tonsillectomy has ranged from a low of 8 percent in one hospital market to a high of nearly 70 percent in another.[48]

How can variations in "practice style" on such an astounding scale possibly be accounted for? The most significant factor driving unnecessary surgeries is that the supplier of surgical services is the prime regulator of demand for those services, and no one is evaluating the outcomes for patients of these major decisions for surgical intervention. It should be vividly clear from the foregoing data that, as long as there is no limit to the ratio of surgeons in the population, there is no limit to how high medical costs can rise within the American medical cosmos as it is presently structured. No limit, other than eventual national bankruptcy.

> Given physicians' ability to generate demand for a substantial portion of their services, such growth will complicate both cost control and the quality of care. . . . As Reinhardt emphasized with regard to American cost-control efforts, decreases in one sector may be readily offset by increases elsewhere. In a fee-for-service system, physicians' styles of practice provide sufficient elasticity to buffer most of the marketplace effects which normally impinge upon the increasing doctor-to-population ratio.[49]

Surgeons clearly are the principal villains feeding the inflation of expenditures for medical care, and the stark reality of supply regulating demand is the indisputable means to this undesirable end.

The examples of *high variation* and *very high variation* surgical causes of hospital admission provided by John Wennberg in his 1988 article is enlightening:

High variation:
   Hysterectomy
   Major cardiovascular operations
   Pediatric hernia operations
   Lens operations
   Major joint operations

Very high variation:
   Knee operations
   Transurethral operations
   Uterus and andenexa operations
   Extraocular operations

Misc. ear, nose, and throat operations
Breast biopsy
D & C, conization except for malignancy
T & A operations except for tonsillectomy
Tonsillectomy

During the past two decades, Wennberg has published other studies on the subject of variation in patterns of medical diagnosis and treatment. In each he has presented clear documentation of prevailing patterns of unnecessary surgical interventions occurring in the United States. In 1973, Wennberg reported that "the most striking example [was] . . . tonsillectomy, which (among thirteen 'hospital service areas' in Vermont) varied from a low of 13 per 10,000 persons to a high of 151 per 10,000 persons." Wennberg concluded that this variation of nearly 12 times the rate of tonsillectomies being performed in the high "hospital service area" as compared to the low area was not explained by an outbreak of rare tonsil disease, but chiefly by variations in "practice style" among ENT surgeons in the two different areas; and by the proportion of ENT surgeons-to-population practicing in these different areas.[50] In 1988, Dr. Wennberg published a "Special Communication" in the *Journal of the American Medical Association (JAMA)* on significant geographic variation in the incidence of prostatectomy for benign urinary tract obstruction. His article includes the following findings:

The Maine Medical Assessment Program provided a forum for discussion of differences in practice styles and the underlying clinical theories. Among Maine urologists, the major controversies about prostatectomy concerned the likelihood for symptom relief and complications following the operation as well as the reasons for performing it in patients without evidence of chronic obstruction. Some physicians advocate surgical intervention in such patients, believing that life expectancy is improved by avoiding the need for operation at a later date. Other physicians believe that the operation does not extend life expectancy in patients without obstruction. They reason that the competing causes of death, the relatively low risk of significant chronic obstruction, and death associated with the operation even in younger patients together mean that the initial loss in life expectancy due to the operation is never regained. . . . The decision analysis indicated that surgery does not prevent death in men without chronic obstruction. In fact, because of the risk of postoperative death, prostatectomy results in a decrease of average life expectancy, and the net benefits of surgery derive from improvement in the quality of life associated with symptom reduction. The analysis thereby highlights the importance of identifying patients' preferences for outcomes that may variably influence their perceptions of the quality of life. Our assessment leads us to conclude that in patients with symptomatic prostatism a randomized trial of prostatectomy vs. watchful waiting would not show definitively which strategy is preferable. . . . The clinical sources of unwanted variations in prostatectomy rates appear to be due to a lack of information concerning the risks and benefits of the procedure, an inappropriate belief that the operation prolongs life, and a failure to base decisions on patient preference for outcomes. We believe that the remedy entails continually improving information on the probabilities of important outcomes and thereby ensuring informed patient decision making, so that decisions are based on patients' attitudes toward risk and their feelings about the various expected outcomes either with or without surgery. We therefore recommend the development of procedures for objectively conveying information to patients about the options open to them in choosing a treatment for prostatic hypertrophy. . . . As one example of this approach, our assessment team is developing an interactive, computer-driven, video disk device to help patients choose between prostatectomy and watchful waiting. The device presents information on the probabilities of outcomes associated with watchful waiting and the operation, and videotaped interviews made of actual patients who have had the operation or elected watchful waiting help the patient understand the significance of the various outcomes . . . there are (other) situations where the objective of a surgical procedure proves to be the reduction of symptoms and the improvement in the quality of life. Many operations appear to fit this class. For example, among the Medicare population, coronary bypass operations, angioplasty, cholecystectomy, hysterectomy, peripheral vascular surgery, total knee and hip replacement, and lens extraction stand out as operations where the primary (if not the exclusive) objective is the improvement of the quality of life. Strategies similar to those we developed in the assessment of prostatectomy may be particularly appropriate for evaluating these procedures.[51]

In 1991 a Wennberg editorial appeared in *JAMA* on the subject of "Unwanted Variations in the Rules of Practice." The following quotations are from that editorial:

Unwanted, practice-style-driven variations in the use of medical care effect underlying confusion over questions of treatment outcomes and the entanglement of the preferences of patients with those of the suppliers and regulators. . . . Practice guidelines need to be based on the methods of science and utilized in a fashion that ensures that patients' preferences are paramount in the choices among plausible treatment options. . . . When well done, the process of constructing guidelines will reveal the many unsettled controversies concerning the effects of treatments on outcomes. In a scientific approach, these identified uncertainties should become the basis for defining priorities for outcomes research. The processes of setting practice guidelines and performing outcomes research are thus related; together they form an ongoing strategy to improve the scientific basis of clinical decision making . . . a consultation with Webster suggests confusion in the debate over practice guidelines. When something is appropriate, it is "especially suitable or compatible," or "fitting." For the many treatments where options exist, third-party guidelines should not prescribe the specific treatment a patient ought to get. The ethical status of the doctor-patient relationship requires that patients be informed about options, that patients' preferences, and not the preferences of their physicians, their employers, or the government, are paramount in the decision to treat. The appropriate use of guidelines requires that they be based on sound science and serve the ethical purpose of making the significance of choice clear to physicians and their patients . . . Practice Guidelines should focus on informing about all reasonable options available for a given condition. In the case of carotid artery stenosis, for example, practice guidelines should be concerned with the outcomes for patients who take aspirin as well as those who elect surgery. Practice guidelines should address all of the outcomes that are relevant to the patient, the risks as well as the benefits, with their probabilities estimated according to the patient's characteristics and treatment chosen. . . . Medical decision making is as much about values and preferences for outcomes as it is about their probabilities. Patients differ in their attitudes toward risk and their preferences for outcomes, and, therefore, in the treatment they consider appropriate for themselves. Many of the conditions for which guidelines are now being developed have more than one "appropriate" treatment. For example, the treatment options for benign prostatic hypertrophy [enlarged prostrate] include surgery, watchful waiting, and, probably very soon, drugs and balloon dilation and, perhaps, even microwave diathermy. Our assessment of alternative treatments of benign prostatic hypertrophy taught us that patients' preferences for treatment cannot be determined by taking a medical history, by performing a physical examination, by testing the flow of urine, or even by asking patients about their symptoms. To know what patients want, patients must be asked in ways that make the options, and uncertainties, clear to them.[52]

In his writings about medical care in the New England states, Wennberg has called attention to another significant but often overlooked fact: the distribution of high-tech medical equipment used in diagnosis and in treatment is often such that the volume of tests or procedures required to maintain the technical proficiency of the physicians and other personnel involved in administering the tests or procedures is absent. For example, the effective use of a linear accelerator in radiation therapy requires that a certain volume of patients are regularly being treated by the radiation therapy team, in order that team members maintain the appropriate level of technical proficiency. In metropolitan statistical areas within New England in which the resident population would need, or would justify, having one such unit, Dr. Wennberg reported finding as many as five in place and in operation. Competing hospitals and competing medical groups have established diagnostic and treatment capacities which are so far in excess of what is necessary and appropriate that in some areas there is no instance in which the patient volume prerequisite to quality medical performance will be available. This is not only wasteful but is also unsafe in that, in the example given, the patient who needs radiation therapy can only receive it from a team of therapists and dosemetrists who lack the required level of technical proficiency because they lack the volume of experience in performing the procedures that is necessary in order to maintain full technical proficiency. The problem is by no means limited to New England; there are thousands of such examples around the nation today.

Situations like these offer additional hard evidence that the scheme of ideas that lies at the base of contemporary medical epistemology is laced with erroneous assumptions and perverse principles. These assumptions and principles go largely unacknowledged within the medical profession, in part because they are never made an explicit part either of formal medical inquiry, or of informal medical dialogue. As a result, the medical profession has generally found it impossible to criticize the foundations, the certitudes, and the presuppositions of its own fundamental thinking. This irreducible reality gives rise to the distinct possibility that American medicine, insofar as it remains blind to the most stubborn facts about the outcomes of its prevailing scheme of ideas, may prove itself to be beyond epistemological redemption or reform.

A Ray of Hope Amid Intimations of Disaster

Leslie L. Roos, professor of management in medicine at the University of Manitoba, also serves as a National Health Scientist for the government of Canada. In 1988, Dr. Roos published an essay entitled "What Does the Future Hold" in *Surgical Care in the United States: A Policy Perspective*. A ray of hope may be discerned within the following paragraphs from Roos's essay: that the interminable trouble with the scheme of ideas influencing the present course of specialization in medicine, rooted as it is in an erroneous cosmology imported from the seventeenth century, might be corrected and redirected.

> Tomorrow's physiology will no longer look like classical physiology, with its boundaries between disciplines within which the function of different organs—including the immune or cardiovascular systems, the kidneys or the brain—was the object of separate studies conducted by different groups that rarely communicated with each other. . . . With a renovated representation of physiological processes, we will gradually move from the traditional approach to life sciences—inducing rules on the basis of experience—to an approach where facts are compared with theory. This development will in turn make it possible to deduce an increasing number of applications—medical, pharmaceutical, and industrial—from theory, whereas today the applications of biology are still often empirical. A more axiomatic context will also transform the way we interpret pathology and make us look for the initial causes, sometimes global, of impaired health. With less fragmented objects of scientific study—organs or functions— and a common language to describe them, the major medical problems will help put into perspective the data accumulated by biological science. It will be possible to mobilize all the resources of theory to answer the challenges of disease in configurations that will be based more on the nature of particular pathological problems than on splitting them up into medical specialties. . . . Universities and institutes of higher learning . . . have not

yet sized up the importance of decompartmentalization in this discipline. Teaching is generally in the mold of the old courses by individual subjects—anatomy, physiology, endocrinology, or immunology—which impedes the widespread adoption of the new "transversal" disciplines that cut across subject lines. Cell biology and molecular genetics are still often taught separately, while they ought to contribute to the restructuring of the traditional fields. What applies to separation into subjects also holds true for career training. Clinical research, pharmaceutical innovation, and thus a good part of medical progress, will depend increasingly on mastering biological axiomatics that are mostly not taught in . . . schools of medicine or pharmacy.[53]

In the meantime, as of the final years of the twentieth century, the stage of evolution which medicine has reached in the United States continues to exhibit, among others, the following undesirable and undeniable characteristics:

- The undergraduate requirements for medical school will no longer include the study of the traditional "liberal arts," such as grammar, rhetoric, logic, mathematics, astronomy, history, and music.

- Graduate medical schools will turn out highly but narrowly trained specialists in large numbers. The brightest of each graduate school class will be rewarded with the prestige of a university faculty appointment. Patients admitted to the university hospital, or to affiliated hospitals, who fall into their specialty or subspecialty will be utilized as teaching material.

- Those who do not do as well in medical school will go into general medicine in solo practice situations, cut off from true engagement with the university world forever. These physicians will take care of the bulk of the medical problems people have, and refer to "specialists" when they feel they are over their heads medically, or when they get into trouble.

- Surgeons will be universally recognized as the dominant players within the university and the hospital. They consistently bring in the largest quantity of federal and other grant dollars; and they consistently contribute the most income from direct medical services and related ancillary services provided to patients. The key measures of financial health for the university hospital will be: How busy are the operating suites? How many operating suites do we have? How busy are the outpatient surgery rooms? How many more of each do we need? Which of the surgical procedures yield the best margins?

- Surgical residencies and other "specialist" fields are presented to medical students as offering the most attractive and the most financially rewarding life for a physician. Medical students who choose a generalist field of practice are considered lacking in the "right stuff," and often view themselves in a similar vein.

- Chiefly as a gesture to federal policy during the 1970s, many university medical schools added residencies in Family Practice within the departments of medicine, however only by recognizing it as a "specialty." Clearly, the same old attitude persists—the generalist is not welcome as an active participant in the medical community of inquiry as it is currently structured in the university setting.

- All financial incentives for physicians will be based on the treatment of sickness or injury, and there will be no way in which any provider of medical services can benefit from health in their patients.

- The supply of physicians will be the major determining factor regulating the demand for medical services. This will be especially true in the variety of surgical fields of practice. The incidence of surgical interventions can, consequently, vary by factors of fifteen times or more from one locale to another, based upon the supply of surgeons, their chosen "practice style," and on their need to earn whatever they decide is a "decent" income. The supply of physicians produced by university medical schools will bear no relationship whatever to a demonstrable and legitimate need for physician "specialists" of the variety being turned out.

- Under its prevailing scheme of ideas, graduate medical education is entirely free not only to churn out an ever-increasing oversupply of surgeons at a cost of hundreds of thousands of dollars per surgeon, but also to set them loose to determine their own practices and procedures; to regulate their own utilization; and to establish their own prices. It would be hard to think of a worse scheme.

- It is of no concern to the medical guild or to those responsible for graduate medical education, that the percent of gross domestic product spent on medical care in the United States is two times what Great Britain spends. Nor is it of concern that the United States has been slipping continuously in relative medical outcomes, including comparisons of overall morbidity and mortality statistics.

- More than half of the hospital discharges in the nation continue to reflect a surgical procedure having been done. In Health Maintenance Organizations (HMOs) contracting with Medicare, as high as 65 percent of the total Part A and Part B dollars paid to the HMO will be required to cover the cost of just five categories of surgical care, and the related anesthesia. The largest single outlay for the care of senior citizens is for the anesthesia services required for the various surgeries they are being subjected to.

- Recognizing the unlimited potential for profitable inpatient surgeries to be performed, and in spite of the intermittent public policy efforts to hold the line on hospital expansion, as many hospital beds as possible will be built. Contradicting a belief that the number of beds has been declining is an April 1997 HCFA report showing a national total of 884,000 short-stay hospital beds in the year 1975; and a national total of 926,000 short-stay beds in 1996. This increase has occurred despite the concurrent growth of HMOs and "managed care" plans, presumably dedicated to radically decreasing the utilization of acute care beds.

- Physicians will be given every incentive to concentrate in urban population centers, up to the point that there will be five to ten times as many as are needed in some cities.

- General medical practice will concentrate on care for the worried well, since few physicians feel that they can afford to work among that segment of the population that presents the most pathology.

- Any amount of money will be spent on harvesting and transplanting organs, but there will always be 10 or 15 percent of the population who will lack access to routine medical care.

- No one in the medical cosmos will be responsible for anyone else. Individuals will be encouraged to shop for service on a trial-and-error basis, with as little information made available about practicing physicians as can be gotten away with. Physicians in fee-based practice will never have a clear idea about what people they have responsibility for. Patients will often have one visit and disappear. "Established" patients will visit other physicians, then come back on occasion, but keep quiet about the other doctor they have seen.

- Women are particularly noted for having two or three "primary" physicians: one for weight control, one for gynecology, and one for general medical problems. No one will be aware of this except the patient, and no one is likely to ask her.

- All information will be stored in records based on the *source* of medical services, and on the distinction between one medical practitioner and another, e.g., "internal medicine," "cardiology," "urology," "endocrinology," "gynecology," or "oncology." It will be made difficult if not impossible to relate information from different sources to a problem presented by a specific patient at a specific time.

In the American medical care system today, the organization of information has been designed principally by death-defiers who cling to an erroneous scheme of ideas. In most instances, the *source of care* is the key to organizing patient information, particularly for the specialist. Most physicians feel that the information in the medical chart belongs to the doctor, not to the patient. Medical records are usually written on this assumption. The handwriting used by many if not most physicians is not legible to the uninitiated. This undoubtedly goes back to ancient Greece, when even the great Hippocrates recommended use of a "secret language" lest a patient discover something which the physician feels they should not know. There has been some experimentation with problem-oriented medical records, in which all medical information is gathered and recorded with reference to the problems presented by a specific patient, and with all information being stored in a unitary chart. This is in contrast with a chart for gynecology, another for endocrinology, another for cardiology, and so forth, all for the same patient. One reason that excellent memory has traditionally been a crucial yardstick in evaluating students of medicine is that lives can depend upon the ability of the physician to relate information from different sources of medical diagnosis and treatment, which is stored in several different records or parts of a record. Memory may therefore be the critical element in a physician reaching a decision about treatment for a specific patient. This is a tangible weakness in the present approach to managing medical information for the benefit of the patient, a weakness which is totally indefensible in light of the advances made in information technology within the past two decades.

Peter Drucker, who has served as a management consultant to many Fortune 500 companies, and who has coined such terms as "global economy," "postmodern," and "information society," among others, predicted over thirty years ago that the most outstanding feature of the twenty-first century would be "the organization of information." This would become the hallmark that would capture the period as the terms "scientific revolution" and "industrial revolution" have done for centuries past. In many fields of inquiry and enterprise other than medicine, the wisdom of Drucker's observation can be seen in concrete ways. Medicine is the most primitive "science" in these terms, primitive in the most pejorative sense of the word. If no other aspect of "modern" American medicine than its management of patient information is subjected to intelligent evaluation, that would suffice to make it irreducibly certain that medicine in the New World has not as yet had its fruitful revolution—neither as an art nor as a science.

Any reasonable person who reflects on the realities of the contemporary medical care system in the United States must recognize the presence of the foregoing litany of characteristics; and as the result of this recognition, ought to understand that the current "crisis" in American medicine is more profound and quite different in nature than is commonly thought.

Surely, no rational person would plan an approach like this for the service system on which the society depends the most; for the system that annually consumes the largest single portion of the gross domestic product. What is it that we are doing here? And what are the implications for the health status of the population? What are the implications of what we are doing for the long-term economic strength of the society? It is clear, at the very least, that people are being operated on by the medical profession inappropriately and unnecessarily. The harm that is currently being done by physicians poses a dilemma for the honest observer: on the scale from vicious to stupid, where should the observer locate physician behavior such as the unnecessary removal of tonsils from a child, or the unnecessary removal of a uterus from a woman, or the unnecessary removal of a prostate gland from a man?

As noted previously, it is an established truth that the outstanding American achievements in "population medicine"—in discovering and implementing effective sanitation and public health measures—are what has enabled American physicians to claim for themselves the title of "world's best medicine." The significant improvements in the health status of the population in the United States have all resulted from innovative public health measures. Except for physician-administered immunizations, the improvements in American health status have had absolutely nothing to do with individual physicians treating individual patients. All of the breakthroughs that have demonstrably improved overall health status have resulted from developments in biomedical science: vaccines and immunizations; improved sanitation; inspection of meat, dairy, and other food products; purification of water supplies; and effective pest control and waste management. It is profoundly ironic that the "top guns" of contemporary American medicine lack any other scientific, medical, or statistical basis upon which to stake their claim to having the "best medical care in the world," and have no other basis—scientific, medical or statistical—on which to legitimately defend themselves against the finding that the medical and surgical services being provided in the United States today include a large measure of the very worst medical care in the world.

This brute fact has not in the slightest way deterred the free barons who control graduate medical education from relegating the limited course material on public health or population medicine contained in medical school curricula to the status of a necessary but unpleasant task, usually presented by the most boring lecturer available.

A Fatally Flawed Scheme

The prevailing scheme of ideas in American medicine, imported from the seventeenth century, has been preventing the medical profession in this country from recognizing and adjusting to the fact that the nature of illness and disease has changed. Medicine is rarely called upon today to deal with episodes of infectious disease. The basic public health measures have been in place for years, although complex new environmental factors are raising new and difficult challenges in population medicine. Rather than dramatic victories over death by the surgical "top guns," however, the real need confronting American medicine is to learn how to intervene in and effectively manage a *process of care* in patients with chronic and degenerative diseases. To the extent that the medical cosmos in the United States today includes process people, they get very little if any recognition, and far less economic reward than the specialists. Nutritional and biochemical scientists form the very bottom of the medical totem, if they are included at all. Consider *diabetes mellitus,* for example: it is probably the most manageable of the leading chronic diseases. If blood sugar levels are carefully and consistently controlled, the disease progresses very slowly and people live with it into their eighties or longer, without the loss of limbs. If the disease is not effectively managed, it will lead to all sorts of expensive complications—amputations, kidney dialysis, cardiovascular disease, blindness—and to premature death. Diabetic patients who understand their disease, and who are provided with the tools necessary to monitor their blood sugar levels several times daily, will rarely if ever require hospitalization for diabetes care. However, at the present time, 68 percent of all the dollars spent annually on the care of diabetics is being spent on inpatient care. The most common admitting diagnosis for these patients is "diabetes out of control." Ninety-five percent of diabetes mellitus patients are managed by their primary-care physician; however, these doctors do not know much about the processes of this disease, or about how to cope with them. Many of the most effective methods and standards for managing diabetes have been developed within the past four or five years, so that 90 percent of the active primary doctors never learned about them in medical school. At the dawn of the twenty-first century, newly diagnosed diabetics are being given the following medical advice by their physicians: "Take this pill every morning, and don't eat sugar." Such behavior gives rise to the question: Does medical care have anything to do with health? Patients are not being taught about their disease because the prospective teacher—the primary doctor— either does not know what or how to teach, or lacks the time or the inclination to do so. Once again, it is impossible to earn a living in the practice of medicine in this country by preventing episodes of illness or disability. With the exception of immunizations, health insurers do not reimburse physicians for interventions aimed at preventing illness and promoting health. Physicians generally have no way to bill their patients for such services. Income for the physician requires a supply of patients who are sick, disabled, or injured. Studies of the ways in which many diabetics are being medically managed by primary physicians in the United States today strongly suggest that much of what is being done might meet the definition of malpractice. Dismissing a diabetic patient from a visit which revealed blood sugars above 400, and telling the nurse to give that patient a return visit weeks or months later, can be seen as totally ridiculous behavior, except when it is considered from the cynical viewpoint of maximizing income in a busy practice.

The predominant mind-set among physicians in the United States is one that steadfastly resists change. If it wasn't learned in medical school, it can't be true. The current medical epistemology produces physicians who find it difficult to accept new knowledge which conflicts in any way with its prevailing, erroneous scheme of ideas. There are many examples, including recent ones, of resistance to and outright rejection of "real" medical science by the free barons of American medicine. The ten-year resistance to Barry Marshall's discovery of *helicobacter pylori* bacteria as the cause of stomach ulcers is a good example. Authority must prevail over experience: shades of the reaction to a new cosmology by the intelligentsia of the seventeenth century. Here we have the identical attitude: when you have a clockwork universe in which all of the parts have been designed and put into place by a supposed master clockmaker, there is no place for new information or new knowledge. It is merely a question of understanding the works in intricate detail, including everything that might go wrong. Once this information has been mastered and committed to memory, learning something new is out of the question. Barry Marshall had simply not accepted the well-established truism in medicine that bacteria cannot live in the "sterile environment" of the human stomach.

Most people would probably think and expect that American physicians in 1983 would greet a discovery like Barry Marshall's with unabated enthusiasm and celebration, not with kicking and screaming. Instead of curiosity, there is the chronic refusal to look again, to reconsider prevailing assumptions, or to reorder traditional logic when new information surfaces. These characteristics would be entirely foreign to the *central vision* on which contemporary scientific inquiry *outside the field of medicine* is based.

It must be recognized, however, that in the ten years during which the *H. pylori* bacteria, although proven as the cause of ulcers, was being overlooked by physicians in the United States, a lot of ulcer surgery took place, surgery that was inappropriate and unnecessary. And a lot of money was spent on that surgery, a goodly portion of which found its way into the pockets of the surgeons, not to mention the psychiatrists and psychologists, who also had an undeserved ten-year supply of patients with ulcer disease. Or the sale of Zantac, the drug of choice for most physicians at the time, at $3 billion per year.

The loss of the generalist mind-set in university medical schools deprives these institutions of the ability to carry on a full-blown and scientifically valid course of medical inquiry. This largely explains the virtual absence of evaluative clinical science in American medicine today—a gap in the armor of the medical free barons that their colleague, John Wennberg, has been warning about for more than a decade. In America, anything can become an accepted medical practice, and usually does.

One look at the comparative statistics on the variation between surgical procedures being performed in the United States and those being performed in Canada is enough to set the mind reeling. For example, the latest report by the American Heart Association (AHA) states that, "In the United States in 1995 an estimated 573,000 CABG (coronary artery bypass surgery) procedures were performed" for a population of 250 million, resulting in a rate of 229.2 procedures per 100,000 citizens. The AHA reports that 74 percent of these procedures were performed on men. An article by Dr. Jane Gentleman in the *Canadian Journal of Surgery* for October 1996 classifies CABG surgery as "intermediate," falling between "primarily discretionary" surgeries such as tonsillectomies and "primarily nondiscretionary" surgeries such as emergency appendectomies. She reports the rate of CABG surgery for Canada's population of 30 million as being 47.4 per 100,000. Thus, the U.S.

rate is nearly five times higher than the Canadian rate for the procedure of which the internationally renowned Dr. Christian Barnard has said: "There is no other operation in the treatment of heart disease more misused than coronary artery surgery. You can earn a lot as a coronary artery surgeon. . . . I would predict that if coronary artery surgery were made illegal in the world today, half the heart surgeons would be out of business and would have to beg for their money, because they exist on this type of surgery." Consider next the variation in a procedure called Carotid Endarterectomy, which has been the subject of controversy in American medical journals. The same two sources report as follows: a 1995 rate of 288.8 per 100,000 in the United States, as compared with a Canadian rate of 8.2 per 100,000. The rate at which this surgical procedure is performed in the United States is more than thirty-five times higher than the Canadian rate. Or take PTCA procedures (Percutaneous Transluminal Coronary Angioplasty), which occurred at a rate of 167.6 per 100,000 in the U.S., with 419,000 procedures being performed during 1995. In Canada, these same PTCA procedures did not make it into the top forty surgical procedures listed by the Health Statistics Division of Statistics Canada, in Ottawa.

The high-technology procedures which "modern" medicine employs, in order to relieve pain or "improve lifestyle" for patients with a disease or disability which physicians do not understand well enough to either cure or prevent, have been misconstrued by the free barons as being real medical science, having something to do with the prevention of illness and the preservation of health in their patients. These high-technology procedures have spawned huge commercial industries, some of them financed through public offerings. When biomedical science discovers a cure for cancer—perhaps in the form of a lovely, individualized vaccine—the situation will be quite different from Sister Kenny's eleemysonary structure, which was shut down overnight without a shareholder's meeting or anything of the sort. There is a legitimate and rather frightening question as to whether, once a cure for cancer has been found, the implementation of it would be impeded by the huge industry which exists in America today, an industry that would be destroyed by real medical science discovering a vaccine-based cure.

Medical leaders in the United States have been supposing that, since the implementation of Flexner's reforms, everything wrong with medicine in America had been fixed. Since this is quite clearly not the case, the logical next question is: What should be done to address these problems? Abraham Flexner was astute enough to issue a warning about the future as a part of his report. He admonished the readers of his report that all of its recommendations would have to be reconsidered in the light of changed conditions within twenty, or at most thirty years. Flexner also believed strongly that there should be no place for "commercialism" in medicine. Flexner's report includes these words:

> In modern life the medical profession is an organ differentiated by society for its own highest purposes, not as a business to be exploited by individuals according to their own fancy. There would be no more vigorous campaigns led by enlightened practitioners against tuberculosis, malaria, and diphtheria, *if the commercial point of view were tolerable in practice.*[54] (Emphasis added)

On the threshold of the twenty-first century, the "commercial point of view" has become not only tolerable, but predominant in American medicine, and the free barons have given ample evidence of the intent to defend that point of view at all cost.

It is interesting to note that tuberculosis, malaria, and diphtheria—all of which had been under effective control on this globe—have all become increasingly prevalent in recent years. Since 1997, many reports have appeared in the medical literature about the renewed virulence of pathogens, evident in hospitals as well as in the general community. The usual assumption in these reports has been that increases in pathogen virulence have resulted solely from an unrestricted and even careless use of antibiotics, leading to a growth in resistance to these drugs on the part of the bacterial pathogens and other parasites. Paul Ewald, a professor in the Department of Biology at Amherst College, has been warning the field of medicine that it must abandon these traditional views on the issue of pathogen virulence, and recognize that increased virulence is occurring because physicians and others who attend to patients have become "cultural vectors," performing the function of "a swarm of mosquitoes" in transmitting pathogens from an immobilized patient to mobile and susceptible hosts. The pathogen infecting an immobilized patient is not in a "survival of the fittest" mode, because survival for it would be impossible if the infection kills off the host. Under these circumstances, pathogens adapt their virulence to suit the situation. However, if physicians and other hospital staff function as "cultural vectors" for the pathogen, survival without the immobile host becomes not only possible, but an avenue for unlimited propagation of the pathogen in mobile, suscep- tible hosts is also opened up. The mechanistic mind-set of most physicians works against the likelihood of easily arriving at this kind of an under- standing of the evolution of pathogen virulence occurring today. Paul Ewald has said the following:

> Without an evolutionary framework for understanding pathogen virulence, researchers would have no reason for expecting to find particularly virulent endemic pathogens in hospitals . . . virulence is positively associated with . . . attendant-borne transmission. . . . Harmful, often antibiotic-resistant, hospital-acquired pathogens can readily emerge beyond a hospital's boundary, when patients are moved, or attendants move between hospitals; the documentation is particularly strong for dangerous variants of E. coli. . . . When large-scale community-wide epidemics of pathogenic E. coli have occurred, for example, transmission in hospitals was strongly implicated. . . . The long-term consequences of emergence of nosocomial strains for the outside community, however, still need to be assessed. The possibility that nosocomial pathogens may tend to be not only more resistant to antibiotics, but also more inherently virulent lends some urgency to this need."

As one of the most mobile and engaged players in the universe of hos- pital attendants, physicians ought to be extremely aware of and concerned about the implications of a rapid evolution of pathogen virulence. Yet, as has been previously noted, despite continuous reminders to them, only 40 per- cent of physicians today comply with their own established protocols for proper hand washing in the inpatient setting. An even smaller percentage keep their stethoscopes clean.

It would be difficult to find in today's literature a more coincidental set of arguments than Ewald's to support my own contention that contemporary medicine has gone astray because of the inadequacies of its intellectual underpinnings and the erroneous content of its dominant "scheme of ideas." Ewald has correctly observed that the "traditional view" of medicine serves to increase the uncertainty about managing the dangerous epidemics of the future. His angle of vision on where the medical field must look for a cor- rection of its traditional views may be discerned from the subtitle of one of his recent articles: "Guarding Against the Most Dangerous Emerging Pathogens: Insights from Evolutionary Biology."

Capability and Willingness?

Here and now, on the eve of the new millennium, the work of reconstruction in medical science, medical education, and medical practice will prove to be not practically possible in the absence of a rigorous and thoroughgoing analysis and reconstruction of the scheme of ideas on which American medical inquiry and practice are currently founded. The cosmology that should drive medical science in the late twentieth century and into the twenty-first century is one derived from Darwin and from Einstein, the scheme of ideas that drives every other legitimate field of scientific inquiry except medicine. This "scheme" postulates a cosmos that is organic, process-oriented, random, and expanding—a multiverse evidently without limits, continuously reminding every serious observer that humanity has but scratched the surface of possible knowledge. Its adherents are driven by curiosity, and are thrilled by discovery.

In order to find its way out of the intellectual box canyon it has gotten itself into, American medicine needs to radically revise and reconstruct its scheme of ideas, using insights drawn from a period which astronomers are now calling the "golden age of cosmology." The pivotal questions are:

(a) Are any of the free barons of American medicine capable of meeting this daunting challenge?

and,

(b) Are any of them willing to make the effort?

Notes

1. K. Popper, *The Logic of Scientific Discovery* (London: Hutchinson, 1958), preface.

2. A. N. Whitehead, *The Function of Reason* (Boston: Beacon Press, 1958), pp. 76–77.

3. A. N. Whitehead, *Process and Reality* (New York: Free Press, 1969), preface.

4. Hippocrates, "Physicians Oath."

5. A. Enthoven, "Managed Competition in Health Care Financing and Delivering: History, Theory, and Practice" (revised paper presented at a workshop sponsored by the Robert Wood Johnson Foundation, Washington, D.C., January 7–8, 1993), p. 2.

6. R. Stevens, *American Medicine and the Public Interest* (New Haven, Conn.: Yale University Press, 1971), p. 30.

7. D. Boorstin, *The Discoverers* (New York: Random House, 1983), p. 71.

8. Ibid., p. 378.

9. H. Butterfield, "Dante's View of the Universe," in *A Short History of Science* (Garden City, N.Y.: Anchor Books, n.d.), pp. 58–59.

10. E. A. Burtt, *Metaphysical Foundations of Modern Physical Science* (Atlantic Heights, N.J.: Humanities Press, 1989), pp. 236–37.

11. T. McKeown, cf. "On the Limitations of Modern Medicine," in J. Powles, *Science, Medicine and Man* (Oxford: Pergamon Press, 1973), p. 13.

12. R. J. Carlson, *The End of Medicine* (New York: John Wiley & Sons, 1975), pp. 202–203.

13. F. S. Taylor, "Scientific Developments of the Early Nineteenth Century," in *A Short History of Science*, p. 83.

14. J. Richmond, *Currents in American Medicine* (Cambridge, Mass.: Harvard University Press, 1969), pp. 1–2.

15. A. N. Whitehead, *Science and the Modern World* (New York: Free Press, 1957), pp. 54–55.

16. Whitehead, *Process and Reality*, p. 241.

17. Ibid., p. 242.

18. J. Robbins, *Reclaiming Our Health* (Tiburon, Calif.: H. J. Kramer, 1996), pp. 16–17.

19. R. Porter, *The Greatest Benefit to Mankind: A Medical History of Humanity* (New York: W. W. Norton, 1997), p. 680.

20. J. Thorwald, *Century of the Surgeon* (New York: Pantheon Books, 1957), p. 227.

21. Ibid., p. 189.

22. J. Randers-Pehrson, *The Surgeon's Glove* (Springfield, Ill.: Thomas Publishing, 1960), p. 21.

23. Ibid., p. 60.

24. Ibid., pp. 61–62.

25. K. Griffin, "They Should Have Washed Their Hands," *Health* (November/December 1996): 82–90.

26. National Center for Health Statistics, "Surgical Procedures" Q&A, from *Advance Data from Vital and Health Statistics*, 1995 Summary National Hospital Discharge Survey (NCHS).

27. Centers for Disease Control Report, "Hospital Infections Program," on-line report on nosocomial infections, at www.cdc.gov/ncidod/publications. Downloaded on May 8, 1998.

28. Centers for Disease Control Report, Summary, Nosocomial Infection Surveillance, 1984, William R. Jarvis et al. Web page converted by CDC April 2, 1998.

29. M. L. Hulsebus, Report commissioned by Board of Medical Device Technologies Inc., chaired by M. Lee Hulsebus: "Latex Surgical Gloves Routinely Fail, Risk of Infection Greater than Believed," published in *Doctor's Guide to Medical News*, March 20, 1997.

30. T. Monmaney, "Marshall's Hunch," *New Yorker*, September 20, 1993, pp. 64–65.

31. Ibid., p. 69.

32. Ibid., p. 72.

33. L. Thomas, *The Lives of a Cell* (New York: Bantam Books, 1975), pp. 35–42:

Technology assessment has become a routine exercise for the scientific enterprises on which the country is obliged to spend vast sums for its needs. Brainy committees are continually evaluating the effectiveness and cost of doing various things in space, defense, energy, transportation, and the like, to give advice about prudent investments for the future.

Somehow medicine, for all the $80-odd billion that it is said to cost the nation, has not yet come in for much of this analytical treatment. It seems taken for granted that the technology of medicine simply exists, take it or leave it, and the only major technologic problem which policy-makers are interested in is how to deliver today's kind of health care, with equity, to all the people.

When, as is bound to happen sooner or later, the analysts get around to the technology of medicine itself, they will have to face the problem of measuring the relative cost and effectiveness of all the things that are done in the management of disease. They make their living at this kind of thing, and I wish them well, but I imagine they will have a bewildering time. For one thing, our methods of managing disease are constantly changing— partly under the influence of new bits of information brought in from all corners of biologic science. At the same time, a great many things are done that are not so closely related to science, some not related at all.

In fact, there are three quite different levels of technology in medicine, so unlike each other as to seem altogether different undertakings. Practitioners of medicine and the analysts will be in trouble if they are not kept separate.

1. First of all, there is a large body of what might be termed "non-technology," impossible to measure in terms of its capacity to alter either the natural course of diseases or its eventual outcome. A great deal of money is spent on this. It is valued highly by the professionals as well as the patients. It consists of what is sometimes called "supportive therapy." It tides patients over through diseases that are not, by and large, understood. It is what is meant by the phrases "caring for" and "standing by." It is indispensible. It is not, however, a technology in any real sense, since it does not involve measures directed at the underlying mechanism of disease.

It includes the large part of any good doctor's time that is taken up with simply providing reassurance, explaining to patients who fear that they have contracted one or another lethal disease that they are, in fact, quite healthy.

It is what physicians used to be engaged in at the bedside of patients with diphtheria, meningitis, poliomyelitis, lobar pneumonia, and all the rest of the infectious diseases that have since come under control.

It is what physicians must now do for patients with intractable cancer, severe rheumatoid arthritis, multiple sclerosis, stroke, and advanced cirrhosis. One can think of at least twenty major diseases that require this kind of supportive medical care because of the absence of an effective technology. I would include a large amount of what is called mental disease, and most varieties of cancer, in this category.

The cost of this nontechnology is very high, and getting higher all the time. It requires not only a great deal of time but also very hard effort and skill on the part of physicians; only the very best of doctors are good at coping with this kind of defeat. It also involves long periods of hospitalization, lots of nursing, lots of involvement of nonmedical professionals in and out of the hospital. It represents, in short, a substantial segment of today's expenditures for health.

2. At the next level up is a kind of technology best termed "halfway technology." This represents the kinds of things that must be done after the fact, in efforts to compensate for the incapacitating effects of certain diseases whose course one is unable to do very much about. It is a technology designed to make up for disease, or to postpone death.

The outstanding examples in recent years are the transplantation of hearts, kidneys, livers, and other organs, and the equally spectacular inventions of artificial organs. In the public mind, this kind of technology has come to seem like the equivalent of the high technologies of the physical sciences. The media tend to present each new procedure as though it represented a breakthrough and therapeutic triumph, instead of the makeshift that it really is.

In fact, this level of technology is, by its nature, at the same time highly sophisticated and profoundly primitive. It is the kind of thing that one must continue to do until there is a genuine understanding of the mechanisms involved in disease. In chronic *glomerulonephritis*, for example, a much clearer insight will be needed into the events leading to the destruction of *glomeruli* by the *immunologic reactants* that now appear to govern this disease, before one will know how to intervene intelligently to prevent the process, or turn it around. But when this level of understanding has been reached, the technology of kidney replacement will not much be needed and should no longer pose the huge problems of logistics, cost, and ethics that it poses today.

An extremely complex and costly technology for the management of coronary heart disease has evolved—involving specialized ambulances and hospital units, all kinds of electronic gadgetry, and whole platoons of new professional personnel—to deal with the end results of coronary thrombosis. Almost everything offered today for the treatment of heart disease is at this level of technology, with the transplanted and artificial hearts as ultimate examples. When enough has been learned to know what really goes wrong in heart disease, one ought to be in a position to figure out ways to prevent or reverse the process, and when this happens the current elaborate technology will probably be set to one side.

Much of what is done in the treatment of cancer, by surgery, irradiation, and chemotherapy, represents halfway technology in the sense that these measures are directed at the existence of already established cancer cells, but not at the mechanisms by which cells become *neoplastic*.

It is a characteristic of this kind of technology that it costs an enormous amount of money and requires a continuing expansion of hospital facilities. There is no end to the need for new, highly trained people to run the enterprise. And there is really no way out of this, at the present state of knowledge. If the installation of specialized coronary-care units can result in the extension of life for only a few patients with coronary disease (and there is no question that this technology is effective in a few cases), it seems to me an inevitable fact of life that as many of these as can be will be put together, and as much money as can be found will be spent. I do not see that anyone has much choice in this. The only thing that can move medicine away from this level of technology is new information, and the only imaginable source of this information is research.

3. The third type of technology is the kind that is so effective that it seems to attract the least public notice; it has come to be taken for granted. This is the genuinely decisive technology of modern medicine, exemplified best by modern methods for immunization against diphtheria, pertussis, and the childhood virus diseases, and the contemporary use of antibiotics and chemotherapy for bacterial infections. The capacity to deal effectively with syphilis and tuberculosis represents a milestone in human endeavor, even though full use of this potential has not yet been made. And there are, of course, other examples: the treatment of endocrinologic disorders with appropriate hormones, the prevention of hemolytic disease of the newborn, the treatment and prevention of various nutritional disorders, and perhaps just around the corner the management of Parkinsonism and sickle-cell anemia. There are other examples, and everyone will have his favorite candidates for the list, but the truth is that there are nothing like as many as the public has been led to believe.

The point to be made about this kind of technology—the real high technology of medicine—is that it comes as the result of a genuine understanding of disease mechanisms, and when it becomes available, it is relatively inexpensive, and relatively easy to deliver.

Offhand, I cannot think of any important human disease for which medicine possesses the outright capacity to prevent or cure where the cost of technology is itself a major problem. The price is never as high as the cost of managing the same diseases during the earlier stages of no-technology or halfway technology. If a case of typhoid fever had to be managed today by the best methods of 1935, it would run to a staggering expense. At, say, around fifty days of hospitalization, requiring the most demanding kind of nursing care, with the obsessive concern for details of diet that characterize the therapy of that time, with daily laboratory monitoring, and, on occasion, surgical intervention for abdominal catastrophe, I should think $10,000 would be a conservative estimate for the illness, as contrasted with today's cost of a bottle of chloramphenicol and a day or two of fever. *The halfway technology that was evolving for poliomyelitis in the early 1950s, just before the emergence of the basic research that made the vaccine possible, provides another illustration of the point. Do you remember Sister Kenny, and the cost of those institutions for rehabilitation, with all those ceremonially applied hot fomentations, and the debates about whether the affected limbs should be totally immobilized or kept in passive motion as frequently as possible, and the masses of statistically tormented data mobilized to support one view or the other? It is the cost of that kind of technology, and its relative effectiveness, that must be compared with the cost and effectiveness of the vaccine* (emphasis added).

Pulmonary tuberculosis had similar episodes in its history. There was a sudden enthusiasm for the surgical removal of infected lung tissue in the early 1950s, and elaborate plans were being made for new and expensive installations for major pulmonary surgery in tuberculosis hospitals, and then INH and streptomycin came along and the hospitals themselves were closed up.

It is when physicians are bogged down by their incomplete technologies, by the innumerable things they are obliged to do in medicine when they lack a clear understanding of disease mechanisms, that the deficiencies of the health-care system are most conspicuous. If I were a policy-maker, interested in saving money for health care over the long haul, I would regard it as an act of high prudence to give high priority to a lot more basic research in biologic science. This is the only way to get the full mileage that biology owes to the science of medicine, even though it seems, as used to be said in the days when the phrase still had some meaning, like asking for the moon.

34. Carlson, *The End of Medicine*, p. 21.

35. D. Blumenthal and A. Scheck (eds.), *Improving Clinical Practice: Total Quality Management and the Physician* (San Francisco: Jossey-Bass, 1995), p. 13.

36. A. Flexner, *Medical Education in the United States* (Boston: Updike and Co., 1910), p. 6.

37. Ibid., p. 28.

38. Ibid., p. 20.

39. Ibid., p. 124.

40. Ibid., pp. 143–48.

41. Ibid., p. 176.

42. Ibid., pp. 167–70.

43. Ibid., p. 19.

44. P. Starr, *The Social Transformation of American Medicine* (New York: Basic-Books, 1982), p. 390.

45. R. Pollock, "A Reappraisal of Emerson," *Thought* 32, no. 124 (Spring 1957): 91.

46. M. Millman, *The Unkindest Cut: Life in the Backrooms of Medicine* (New York: Morrow & Co., 1977), p. 231.

47. D. Stroman, *The Quick Knife* (Port Washington, N.Y.: Kennikat Press, 1979), p. 155.

48. J. Wennberg, "Variation in Surgical Practice: A Proposal for Action," in *Surgical Care in the United States: A Policy Perspective*, ed. M. L. Finkel (Baltimore: Johns Hopkins University Press, 1988), p. 61.

49. L. Roos, "What Does the Future Hold?" in Finkel, *Surgical Care in the United States*, p. 177.

50. J. Wennberg, "Small Area Variations in Health Care Delivery," *Science* 182, December 14, 1973, p. 1105.

51. J. Wennberg et al., "An Assessment of Prostatectomy for Benign Urinary Tract Obstruction," *Journal of the American Medical Association* 259 (May 27, 1988): 3027–30.

52. J. Wennberg, "Unwanted Variations in the Rules of Practice," *Journal of the American Medical Association* 265, no. 10 (March 13, 1991): pp. 1306–1307.

53. C. Kordon, *The Language of the Cell* (New York: McGraw-Hill, 1993), pp. 96–97.

54. Flexner, *Medical Education in the United States*, p. 19.

55. P. Ewald, "Guarding Against the Most Dangerous Emerging Pathogens: Insights from Evolutionary Biology," *Emerging Infectious Diseases* 2, no. 4 (October/December 1996): 252–53.

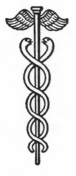

4.

Legislative Remedies
Increase the Illness

The most stubborn, most irreducible fact about the causes
of radical inflation in expenditures for medical and hospital care is that there is a massive oversupply of physicians
practicing in the United States today under a fee-for-service system in which the supplier of medical services—the
physician—is the regulator of demand for the entire range
of services provided to patients. Many people may question whether fee-for-service remains a significant factor in
American medicine, since there has been so much pub-
licity about the growth of HMOs and "managed-care"
plans, which are supposed to pay physicians on a different
basis. Some will argue that the HMO and "managed-care"
plans have radically reduced fee-based payment of physicians. To demonstrate the falsity of this argument, attention is directed to the following relevant facts:

- As indicated in chapter 1, the American Medical
  Association's *AMNews* reported on January 20,
  1997 that the share of *all physician revenue* from *all
  HMO/managed-care contracts* was 27.1 percent of
  total physician revenue. This means that 72.9 percent of all physician revenue came from sources

unrelated to contracts with HMO/managed-care plans. The *AMNews* noted in this report that this 27.1 percent share of all revenue represented a *decrease* from a 34 percent share of all revenue in the previous year, thus a nearly seven-point decline in revenue from these sources had occurred.

- The Interstudy *Competitive Edge* report published in April 1998 includes the following pertinent data. HMO plans were separated into two classes:

     Category I.   Low users of FFS, being those plans that reimburse less than 40 percent of primary MDs on a fee-for-service basis; and,

     Category II.   High users of FFS, being those plans that reimburse more than 40 percent of primary MDs on a fee-for-service basis.

The Interstudy report shows that for the high users of FFS, [HMO] enrollment grew much faster during the 1995–1997 period than it did for the plans that were low users of FFS. The study concludes that "between July 1995 and July 1997, overall [HMO] enrollment growth [nationally] has been driven by fee for service primary care systems." Even more dramatic evidence that fee-for-service is thriving may be seen in the data comparing Categories I & II plans for high and low *capitation* use by HMOs:

     Category I.   Only 19 percent of low users of FFS are high users of capitation; while 11 percent of low users of FFS (mostly plans that salary physicians) are also low users of capitation; and,

     Category II.   Zero percent of high users of FFS are high users of capitation, while 70 percent of high FFS users qualified as low capitation users.

As for specialty care, the Interstudy report includes the following statements: "As with primary care reimbursement, the percent of [HMO] enrollees served by specialty care physicians reimbursed by fee schedules grew considerably between July 1995 and July 1997. The percent of HMOs using fee schedules for specialty care reimbursement is 85 percent, and has remained stable since July 1993." The facts presented here are readily verifiable, and should be sufficient to remove any doubt about the fact that fee-based payment continues to be dominant in American medicine.

Many people may now believe that the HMOs and "managed-care" plans, through their administrative employees, control medical decisions affecting their members, and that they, and not the doctors, are therefore the true regulators of the demand for medical services. During the past five years, the American Medical Association, many practicing physicians, and most hospitals have been waging a clever, progressively more intense and expensive national campaign to convince the society, using the "big lie" technique and the awful anecdote, that the HMO/managed-care plans have taken control of medical decision making. Although this is utter nonsense, and physicians know it, the well-organized campaign has had considerable success in suggesting to the society that there is someone besides licensed physicians out there practicing medicine. The facts, however, are these:

- All states and the federal government have statutes and regulations that prohibit anyone from making a medical decision affecting a patient except for the physician or physicians who are treating that patient. Nurse practitioners and physician assistants must perform their functions under the active supervision of a licensed physician.

- It is axiomatic that no employee of an HMO, whether a licensed physician or not, may legally make a medical decision about the care of a patient, unless they happen to be the attending physician of that patient, which would be a very rare occurrence. No hospital would permit the acceptance of orders or instructions regarding the care and treatment of a patient issued by any other source than that patient's attending physician, or a referral physician who has been formally brought into the case by the attending physician. It simply cannot happen.

- What the national fuss is really all about, despite what the AMA would have us believe, is the interpretation of the variety of *benefits contracts.* When you join a health plan, either a group or an individual contract must be executed, committing all parties to its terms. In the case of an HMO that is a true *direct service* plan, such as the Kaiser Health Plan, the contractual promise is not to pay the bills for medical or hospital care which you go out and arrange for yourself, but rather to use the income from member premiums to set up an organized system of medical and hospital services that will be there when a member needs them, every day; and for emergencies, at all hours, every day.

- The anecdotal "horror stories" being propagated by the medical guild and its allies stem mainly from contract disputes, many of the more dramatic stories having to do with emergency care. For example, there was a story about a woman turned away by the ER at one hospital because her HMO would only pay if she went to the ER the HMO had a contract with, which was twenty miles away. The story was that the woman died before reaching the second ER. If this story were true, the following facts would bear notice:

    1. Every facility that presents itself to society as a provider of emergency medical care must care for every person that presents themselves at the ER with an emergent medical condition.

    2. In all fifty states, it is impermissible to turn any truly emergent case away from a facility that labels itself as an emergency room. The only exception made is for a situation in which a large-scale disaster may have totally overwhelmed the resources of a given ER. The emergency facility may then notify ambulance operators and emergency technicians in the field not to bring cases there until the crisis has been managed. There are no other exceptions, and services for emergent conditions must be provided regardless of a patient's ability to pay. If the ER turned the woman in the aforementioned story away, and if she had a medical emergency, as would seem likely if she then died, the ER doctor who made the decision to deny care is solely and fully responsible, no matter what the doctor may have been told by an HMO administrative person about payment, or about ER contracts, or anything else. The ethical duties and legal responsibilities of emergency-room physicians are crystal clear when it comes to ER care, and the foregoing anecdote, intended to be critical of an HMO, simply does not bear scrutiny.

3. Those who arrive at an ER who do not have an emergent medical condition are in the wrong setting, and should be directed to the proper source of care. Most of the disputes between ER doctors and HMOs concern this category of patient, i.e., a patient who does not require emergency care, although they may be sick or injured. The ER physicians almost always know the pertinent medical facts, however, they would prefer to treat these patients anyway, and bill the insurer for the nonemergency care. For indemnity insurers, this has been the normal and customary pattern, because their contractual responsibility is to pay the bills after the fact for services that the policyholder sought out and obtained for themselves.

- The responsibility of an HMO is quite different, as has been noted above. It is to set up a network or system of direct medical and hospital services consistent with the benefit contracts of its members, and to have those services available to members when they need them. The conflicts that may occur between HMOs and their members are contractual disputes about whether a particular service or benefit is covered under the contract in force. HMOs do not make medical decisions, they only make coverage decisions.

Fee-Based Medicine: Serving Society's Highest Purposes?

If the AMA is telling the society that, unless or until the doctor has gotten a satisfactory guarantee of payment for the services from *someone*, physicians will not provide the care that a patient they are attending is medically in need of, then the American public should fully recognize this entirely commercial point of view on the part of the medical profession, and should fully consider its unsettling implications.

The fact that so-called organized medicine is not happy about the significant changes being gradually introduced by HMOs is evidenced by the aggressive and well-financed campaigns that the medical associations have underway throughout the nation to stop the progress of HMOs and "managed care," and to prevent any further erosion of market share for its still very powerful physician guild. The AMA, seeing the handwriting very clearly on the walls in such "high change" states as California and Minnesota, where HMOs have done well, has launched efforts through its state and county affiliates to undermine and destroy the essential building blocks of an HMO or "managed-care" approach, for example, the ability to contract with a select panel of physicians to provide care to the enrolled members of a health plan. Two bills were introduced in the Florida legislature in the 1995 session, at the behest of the Florida Medical Association and the Dade County Medical Association, with blatantly misleading titles: the "Patient Protection Act" and the "Patient Freedom of Choice Act." These proposed laws would allow any member of an HMO or "managed-care" plan to freely elect to go to any physician they wished to see, at any time, and would require the patient's HMO or "managed-care" organization to pay any physician providing medical services to these members their "usual and customary" fees, in other words, their billed charges. At federal and state levels, the AMA and its affiliates have been pushing a variety of bills under the equally grandiose and misleading heading of "any willing provider." The concept here is that an HMO's members may visit any doctor who is willing to see them, and their HMO has to pay all resulting bills. The effort in these cases has been to pass laws that would deprive HMOs and "managed-care" organizations of the ability to selectively contract with a specific panel of physicians to care for their membership, using the economic power of their membership base to obtain a volume discount from the contracting physicians, in return for assuring the doctors a significant market share (the HMO's members) for their medical practice. The medical guild is well aware of the fact that, if any of these devious and anticompetitive AMA-led efforts should succeed, HMOs and "managed-care" plans would thereby be undermined in ways that would very quickly prove to be fatal.

Unfortunately, most legislators are fair game for these sorts of initiatives by the AMA and its state affiliates. "Organized medicine" has been and is a major source of political contributions at all levels of government, and their legislative proposals virtually always come with a disinformation cover designed to make them sound like the next best thing to motherhood and apple pie. The current medical guild pattern is to undergird these legislative initiatives not only with hard cash, but also by having member physicians appear before legislative committees to testify about the poor quality of care being provided by HMO or "managed-care" physicians, using anecdotes of horror-story caliber to make patently false accusations appear true to the elected officials, and to the general public. Recent examples include the testimony of a dermatologist, speaking on behalf of the Florida Medical Association in support of an "any willing provider" bill, in which he told the story of a patient, *referred to him by an HMO primary-care physician,* whom he diagnosed as having lupus. The dermatologist did not otherwise identify the patient's disease, despite the fact that the term "lupus," used alone, has no specific diagnostic meaning. It must have either the modifier *vulgaris* or the modifier *erythematosus* in order to have a specific medical meaning. The physician knew this, but the legislators did not. Furthermore, there are two forms of *Lupus erythematosus,* one a fairly mild skin disorder, and the other causing deterioration of the connective tissues in various parts of the body, including soft internal organs, bones, and muscles. This latter form of *Lupus erythematosus* is often fatal, and there is no specific treatment for the disease, although there are treatments to provide symptom relief. As the record of his testimony will show, the dermatologist revealed none of these pertinent facts to the committee, or to those in attendance. Everyone was left to conclude that this was the lupus we have heard about, which is usually a slow death sentence for the patient. The dermatologist testified that, in reviewing the history of this patient sent to him by the referring primary doctor, he learned that the chest rash for which the patient was referred had appeared a month or so earlier. He told the committee that he then decided that the rash had been a precursor to lupus, not otherwise defined during the dermatologist's testimony. The dermatologist also informed the committee that he deplored the fact that the patient's HMO primary physician had failed to make the diagnosis of lupus at the time of the initial encounter with the patient. This was presented to the legislators as definitive proof that HMO physicians are not as capable as non-HMO physicians; that primary care physicians are not as capable as "specialists"; and that HMOs represented a barrier to having patients diagnosed appropriately, and on a timely basis. In the real world, however, a competent board-certified family physician may miss making the potential connection between a chest rash and the presence of *Lupus vulgaris*; or of *Lupus erythematosus,* in either of its forms; and so may a board-certified dermatologist, whether the physician in question is in fee-for-service practice, or with an HMO, or both. Most patients with a rash begin with their primary doctor, and not with a dermatologist. As a matter of fact, the primary physician being publicly trashed by the dermatologist that day in Tallahassee had a practice made up of 80 percent non-HMO patients and 20 percent HMO patients, all of them under fee-for-service reimbursement. The members of the Florida state legislative committee, however, concluded at that session—and on the basis of the dermatologist's dramatic testimony—that additional legislative constraints should be imposed on HMOs and "managed-care" plans, to enable members to visit the specialist of their choice for any reason, or for no reason, and requiring the HMO to pay all resulting bills. State law in Florida today provides that any member of an HMO may self-refer to a licensed dermatologist up to five times during any calendar year, without prior authorization from their health plan, and provides that the plan must pay the dermatologist for those services. "Guild Free Choice" won a round in Florida, a relatively "low-change" state in terms of HMO enrollment levels. Dermatology has opened the door; can surgery be far behind?

The Sky Is No Limit

There is another very stubborn and irreducible fact about the radical inflation in medical and hospital outlays that needs to be paid strict attention: given all of the foregoing facts, and as things now operate, no matter what the experts may tell us, there is no way to predict how high overall expenditures for medical and hospital care may rise.

In the thirty-year span from 1965 to 1995, the annual per capita expenditure for medical care in the United States jumped by 2,000 percent, from $204 per person to $4,100 per person. If the same rate of increase occurs during the next thirty years, the annual per capita figure would rise to $82,000—and the nation would be bankrupt. Even if the population remained static, the national expenditure for medical care would be $20 trillion per year—*twenty times* what we are spending today. This is the course that the country is currently pursuing, and despite all of the talk of reform, these most stubborn and most irreducible facts about the causes of this national disaster are being steadfastly ignored by elected officials and public policy makers. Such persistent efforts at ignoring these hard realities can only be explained by the direct and indirect power and influence of the American medical guild. The culture has placed physicians on a pedestal; we still view them as good guys who are dedicated to helping us stay alive. The notion that there are some medical free barons who are in fact the bad guys who now threaten to destroy the national economy is a notion that this culture is ill-prepared to accept, despite the documented proof that many surgical and invasive diagnostic procedures are being performed on innocent people by physicians motivated chiefly by their own greed. What could be worse than to be cut open and victimized by one of these radical rascals when there is no sound medical reason to justify the surgery? Expenditures of $20 trillion per year for medical care may seem too fantastic a projection to be believed, yet even with no increase in the population, annual healthcare expenditures would in fact rise to that level if the pattern during the past thirty years is repeated during the next thirty years.

Consider an alternative question: what ought to be the level of national healthcare expenditures in the United States? The highly respected Pew Health Professions Commission recently reported that the optimal ratio of physicians to population would be 150 per 100,000 persons. They also reported that the nation will be close to twice that ratio by the year 2000—at 290 per 100,000.

- The AMA reported that median physician income in the United States declined to $150,000 in 1995. Adding overhead at 60 percent, the gross figure would be $240,000.
- The AMA has also reported that physicians receive less than twenty cents of each healthcare dollar spent.

For the current U.S. population, the optimal ratio cited in the Pew report would require 375,000 physicians *in toto*. Assuming the AMA median income plus overhead at 60 percent, the total annual outlay for this national physician cadre would be $80 billion.

Assuming that $80 billion represents 20 percent of total expenditures for health care, the correct gross national annual outlay ought to be five times that, or $400 billion. That represents just 40 percent of what is actually being expended today. The difference from actual expenditures is explained chiefly by the stubborn and irreducible facts of a radical and continuously worsening oversupply of physicians working within an economic system in which they are the regulators of their own demand.

The brutal truth is that the culture ignores these stubborn, irreducible realities at its own peril. Ignoring these concrete facts has led the Congress and many state legislatures to enact laws that have mainly served to deepen and worsen the crisis. Over the past thirty-five years, a series of pivotal public policy decisions have tended to make things much worse, in part because each of those decisions has been rooted in assumptions that were erroneous, pernicious, or both. For example, consider the following litany of congressional legislative follies:

1. Hill-Burton (The Hospital Survey and Construction Act of 1946, sponsored by Sen. Lister Hill and Rep. Phillip Burton)
    Erroneous Assumption: There is a shortage of hospital beds.
2. Medicare and Medicaid
    Erroneous Assumption: Pumping more dollars into health care would suffice; no reform of the system would be required.
3. Medical Education
    Erroneous Assumption: The nation had a shortage of physicians, especially in the various "specialties."
4. Medical Research
    Erroneous Assumption: It is not important to distinguish between basic medical science and medical technology.
5. Alphabet Soup: CHP, CMP, CON, DRG, GMENAC, HMA, HSA, PPAC, PPRC, PPS, PRO, PSRO, AND RMP all intended to control the inflation of healthcare costs, but instead they fueled the inflationary fires. (CHP = Comprehensive Health Planning; CMP = Competitive Medical Plan; CON = Certificate of Need; DRG = Diagnosis Related Group; GMENAC = Graduate Medical Education National Advisory Committee; HMA = Health Manpower Act; HSA = Health Services Agency; PPAC = Prospective Payment Assessment Commission; PPRC = Physician Payment Review Commission; PPS = Prospective Payment System; PRO = Peer Review Organization; PSRO = Professional Standards Review Organization; RMP = Regional Medical Program)
    Erroneous Assumptions: There is some purpose to be gained by closing the barn door after the horses have run off; and, dollars alone will cure this grave malady, which threatens the society.

6. FEHBP, CHAMPUS, and AAPCCs (FEHBP = Federal Employees Health Benefits Plan; CHAMPUS = Civilian Health and Medical Program of the Uniformed Services; AAPCC = Adjusted Average Per Capita Cost)
Erroneous Assumption: Federal civil servants will act shrewdly in purchasing health benefits covered by government programs.

This incredible set of erroneous assumptions has caused the Congress to act in ways that have increased the systemic disease with every remedy undertaken. In every instance except one, the laws enacted can correctly be described as making the right thing in medical care very difficult to do, and the wrong thing very easy to do. The overarching legislative assumption, in recognition of the power of the American medical guild, has been that the easiest thing for the Congress would be to head in the direction the horse wanted to go. The great problem with this approach is that, absent divine intervention, it can never get you to where *you* want and need to go.

In what follows I have attempted an examination in some detail of the nature of the assumptions surrounding each of the six foregoing categories of legislative health care initiatives undertaken by the Congress during the past three and a half decades.

Writing in 1969 about hospital regulation in the United States, at a time when the scale of congressional folly in enacting the Hill-Burton Act was becoming clear to health-policy people, Anne R. Somers, the author of *Health Care in Transition: Directions for the Future,* said:

> It is difficult to exaggerate the importance of the hospital in contemporary society. It has become the central institution in the organization and delivery of health services, essential both to the care of the patient and to the practice of medicine. . . . The hospital is to modern America what the cathedral was to Europe in the Middle Ages: a complex social institution serving simultaneously a variety of purposes—welfare center, object of civic pride, major source of employment, market for artists, artisans, and architects, inspirer of saintly deeds and beneficiary of repentant sinners, occasional "cover-up" for hypocrites and exploiters, source of power, and object of political conflict. Both institutions have reflected the values of their day. Both have contained deep internal contradictions. Both have defied conventional public regulation.[1]

It is interesting to note that Somers reached back to the Middle Ages for an analogy to the hospital in contemporary American culture, for the hospital is, after all, the workshop of the physician free barons who have formed the medical guild in America, the roots of which are to be found in medieval Europe.

The prevailing scheme of ideas of the medical guild postulates a clockwork universe that is hospital-centered: virtually every other component in the medical cosmos has been arranged around this center, and has had its actions controlled by the gravitational forces exerted by this central body. Every actor in the world of American medicine has had his or her cosmic significance defined, justified, and accounted for in terms of placement within this hierarchical arrangement.

The hospital is the workshop of the surgeons, and the surgical suites have become the sacristy of this modern cathedral, with the surgeons themselves being treated as God-like high priests, performing their ministrations in the operating theatres, the true inner sanctums of the modern medical cathedral. Those physicians on whom all other physicians must depend for specific diagnostic services, such as radiologists and pathologists, have been permanently situated within the cathedral. The anesthesiologists, on whom all surgeons depend, have been exclusively officed within the hospital. The remainder of generalist and specialist physicians, including the large variety of surgical specialists, have done their best to locate their private offices within hailing distance of the hospital, frequently in a medical office building adjacent to the cosmic center, and on the same "campus." The proximate physical location of doctors to the hospital serves their own convenience, as well as the convenience of the patients who are referred to medical colleagues, or who are admitted as inpatients. This vital center of the American medical cosmos—the hospital—has been under the firm control of physician free barons, the effective "prime movers" within medicine's clockwork universe.

During Harry S. Truman's administration, the United States Congress unwittingly played the role of a *deus ex machina* to this medical cosmos, when it passed the Hospital Survey and Construction Act of 1946—popularly known as the Hill-Burton Act. The act provided the funding for a huge expansion in the number of hospitals in the nation, and in the number of acute-care beds. In 1964, the act was amended to go beyond new construction and include monies for modernization and renovation of existing hospitals. The amended bill was called the Hill-Harris Act. By the time this law expired in 1969, total expenditures for hospital construction, modernization, and renovation exceeded $10 billion. Roughly one-third of the dollars came from the federal treasury, with the balance coming from state and local sources.

As World War II ended, Sen. Lister Hill had shared the then-widespread assumption that the nation was sorely lacking in hospital beds, particularly in the rural areas of the country. There is little evidence of any quibbling with this assumption at the time, and the massive hospital construction program was launched. It has been reliably reported that, during the ensuing twenty-two years, at least one hospital was built under Hill-Burton in every single congressional district in the United States.

According to Rosemary Stevens, in her book *American Medicine and the Public Interest,* during the first twenty years under Hill-Burton and Hill-Harris, 4,678 projects received federal financing, and 425,000 hospital and nursing-home beds were either built anew or modernized. In addition, 2,800 other health facilities were added to the national inventory.[2] The National Center for Health Statistics (NCHS) has reported that, during the period from 1960 to 1975, national health expenditures rose from $25.9 billion to $122.2 billion, an increase of nearly 500 percent, or an average of 31 percent per year. During this same period, based on NCHS statistics, the percentage of total healthcare dollars being spent for hospital care jumped by an astounding 20 percent, from 33 percent of the total dollars in 1960 to 40 percent of total dollars in 1975. This percentage has remained above 40 ever since. The dramatic increase during these years in the number of acute-care hospital beds, a growth of nearly 30 percent, was stimulated chiefly by the policies and the actions of the Congress.

The Congress did not anticipate that, just as massive hospital construction was underway in rural areas of the nation, huge numbers of people in postwar America were deciding to concentrate in urban-suburban metropolitan areas, which were expanded rapidly to meet the demand for new housing, schools and other community resources. This dramatic migration of the population from rural to urban-suburban communities led eventually to the Hill-Harris changes, so that existing urban hospitals could obtain federal financing needed to increase their inventory of acute-care beds, and to modernize existing plant and equipment.

It was Milton Roemer, M.D., who, more than three decades ago, gave us the pertinent maxim about hospital construction: "Hospital beds that are built tend to be used." This has become known as "Roemer's Law." The level of demand for hospital care is totally under the control of physicians: the *essential suppliers* are also the *essential controllers* of the demand for acute-care hospital bed use. Within this medical wonderland, the only effective or practical constraint on the level of demand for acute-care bed utilization is the actual number of hospital beds available.

With the Hill-Burton Act, Congress created a recurring nightmare for the American public. Many irrefutable studies have demonstrated the harm that has been done to innocent people as the result of the radical oversupply of hospital beds produced at the urging of the members of Congress. Where the rate of hospital beds to population is high, so are the rates of such "gray area" surgeries as tonsillectomies, adenoidectomies, and hysterectomies.

As early as 1970, a study in Vermont demonstrated a perverse relationship between hospital utilization rates and infant mortality rates: the higher the former, the higher the latter. This study concluded that the residents of poorer areas of the state used less hospital care per capita—42 percent less use in the case of residents with the lowest median income; and that the infant mortality rate for those with the lowest median income was 55 percent below the infant mortality rate for the residents with the highest median income.

> Infant mortality is often cited as a general indication of the quality of medical care. In Vermont, however, it was found that the poorer areas using less services had relatively lower infant mortality rates. Table 14 shows the rank order of Vermont's 251 towns in terms of their median income placed into 10 groupings with Group 1 containing the towns with the highest incomes and Group 10 the lowest. It also shows infant mortality rates for 1969 for the 10 groupings.

TABLE 14

Rank Order Median Income	Infant Mortality Rate (1968-1970)	Hospital Utilization Rate for 1969
1 (highest)	26.2	193.3
2	16.4	191.7
3	21.5	193.5
4	15.6	201.1
5	21.6	167.5
6	20.4	169.0
7	17.3	154.5
8	17.0	140.4
9	15.7	102.5
10 (lowest)	14.4	82.4

In analyzing this data, high income, high infant mortality and high utilization of hospitals seem to show positive correlations. However, we do not suggest that lower utilization causes lower infant mortality. However, the result is surprising and should be considered further.[3]

It is also surprising that the well-off folks in the Hardwick and Middlebury areas of Vermont, where this study was conducted, may have had the excess-bed capacity created by the U.S. Congress to thank in some measure for the terrible reality that their expectant mothers were being told almost twice as often as the Vermont women from the other side of the tracks that their new-born baby was dead.

Lawrence Williams, M.D., published a book in 1971 entitled *How to Avoid Unnecessary Surgery* in which he compared surgical rates in the United States and Britain:

> [T]here is one operation per year for every thirteen people in the United States. Astonishingly, . . . in England and in Wales, . . . the operations rate per year is only one for every twenty-six people: yes, one-half the rate of the United States. . . . [T]he 20 percent unnecessary surgical rate figure used throughout this book is probably a conservative estimate.[4]

During the same period in which federal financing of hospital construction increased the number of acute-care beds in the United States by 40 percent, the Congress was also busy financing a radical increase in the nation's capacity for producing licensed physicians. An analogous, equally erroneous assumption was at work: that there was a physician shortage in America. We now recognize that there was an inadequate distribution of physicians, and not a shortage. Between 1960 and 1978, Congress provided taxpayer funds to support an increase of 44 percent in the number of medical schools in the United States. Roemer's Law about hospital beds once built tending to be used is equally true of surplus medical doctors. Congress built the beds, and it also built the factories to turn out a huge surplus of physicians who have been actively utilizing those excess beds to their own best advantage.

A compelling argument can be made that the continuous worsening of morbidity and mortality statistics for the American population, as compared with the same statistics for all other industrialized nations of the contemporary world, can be judged the direct result of actions by the U.S. Congress in enacting the Hill-Burton law, and in simultaneously financing a radical expansion of medical school facilities, thereby causing the production of the current radical oversupply of licensed physicians—particularly "specialists."

Oversupply Drives Expenditures

The oversupply of hospital beds, combined with the oversupply of practicing physicians, are two of the root causes of the radical inflation in the level of national expenditures for medical care. An article in the *New York Times* for September 15, 1998, based on a new federal projection of health-expenditure trends, reports that the $1 trillion national annual outlay for medical care will more than double by the year 2007, rising to $2.1 trillion. The report projects increases in spending for physician services at a rate of 8 percent per year between 1999 and 2007. The federal analysts state that "population growth accounts for a relatively small share of the increase in total health spending." As noted in chapter 3, the notion that there has been a steady decline in the inventory of hospital beds is disputed by an April 1997 HCFA report showing a national total of 884,000 short-stay hospital beds in the year 1975, and a national total of 926,000 short-stay beds in 1996. This increase has occurred in spite of the growth of HMOs and "managed-care" plans during this period, presumably resulting in radical decreases in the utilization of acute-care beds. In light of these recent federal reports anticipating the resumption of large annual jumps in total healthcare expenditures, a clear and present threat to the economic health of the nation may now be more readily recognized. Lacking a clear understanding of the workings of the American medical cosmos, or of the structures and the interstices of the medical guild, federal legislators seem to have had no idea that financing radical increases in the supply of acute-care hospital beds and in the supply of physicians would lead as inexorably as it has done to a worsening of the health status of the American people, and to the clear and present threat of national bankruptcy.

The road leading to this particular hell has surely been paved with good intentions on the part of many legislators. However, unless the lessons of the past are fully learned and understood, Congress is bound to repeat and multiply the devastating folly of its previous legislative adventures as it undertakes further efforts to reform the American medical care system. The most pressing lesson is that reconstruction of the current medical cosmos, and of the scheme of ideas that drives it, must precede any further infusion of dollars into medical and health care.

In 1965, when Congress enacted Title XVIII of the Social Security Act, entitled "Health Insurance of the Aged," or Medicare, the legislators decided that medical and hospital services provided to the nation's "senior citizens" would be financed in large part by the federal government.

It is important to remember that, as Paul Starr, a Harvard professor of sociology, has noted in his masterful book *The Social Transformation of American Medicine: The Rise of a Sovereign Profession and the Making of a Vast Industry,* Franklin D. Roosevelt had the idea of universal health care on his New Deal agenda, but never formally proposed it to the Congress because he calculated that the hostile reaction from the medical guild would prove fatal to any such initiative. Starr has recorded the fact that, "Even a discussion of general principles for health insurance . . . aroused a storm of protest from the AMA. . . . [T]he AMA called a special meeting of its House of Delegates in February, 1935—only the second in history—where it once again denounced compulsory health insurance and any lay control of medical benefits in relief agencies."[5] Some of Roosevelt's cabinet members kept pushing the health agenda as a part of New Deal social reforms, and in 1939, Sen. Robert Wagner of New York introduced national health insurance legislation. Starr reports that the AMA opposed the Wagner bill *in toto,* and President Roosevelt then informed the Congress that all he wanted on health was some funds for hospital construction. This most powerful of U.S. presidents fully recognized the overwhelming political clout of the physician free barons of the AMA. In January 1944, in his last State of the Union address, Roosevelt did ask the Congress to declare an "economic bill of rights" that he believed belonged to every American. One of the rights was adequate medical care, and the means to obtain it. Harry Truman became the first president to propose passage of universal health care, and by doing so, he proved the political wisdom of his predecessor. Starr tells us that, a few months after he succeeded Roosevelt as President, Truman formally asked Congress to pass a national program to assure every citizen "the right to adequate medical care and protection from the economic fears of sickness." After Truman was elected in his own right, in the surprise of 1948, Starr observes that: "the AMA thought armageddon had come. It assessed each of its members an additional $25." The AMA's special assessment on its member physicians raised a war chest of $3.5 million to finance the fight against universal health care. The AMA launched a powerful and severely abusive campaign against any federal interference with the practice of medicine, or with the way in which guild members structured the financial rewards for their medical services. "Socialized medicine" became its war cry. Truman waged his own countercampaign, but was eventually faced with the reality that he could not beat the AMA and its lobbyists. The president then looked for a less sweeping alternative to universal health care, and the idea of Medicare was born. Truman had every expectation that the new program, which in 1966 would cover 19 million seniors, would eventually be expanded into a universal health-insurance program.

In 1965, recognition of the political power of the medical guild was such that the initial legislative proposal for Medicare covered only hospital care, and provided no payment for physician services. The intent was to reduce the opposition from the AMA and the free barons of medicine in order to get a health-insurance bill covering seniors passed and signed into law. During the mark-up of the bill by the Ways and Means Committee, Chairman Wilbur Mills added Part B (designed to reimburse physicians for specified services) at the last stages of the legislative process, just about as it stands today. The AMA lobbyists inserted the wording "usual, customary, and reasonable" as the only measuring rod for reimbursement of physician fees; and they also made certain that the only criterion that could be applied to evaluation of the care provided would be whether or not the services were "medically necessary." Of course, only the free barons would be in a position to judge "medical necessity." The initial premium for Part B coverage was $3 from the beneficiary, and $3 from the federal treasury. Enrollment in Part B was, and remains, voluntary. The premium for Part B Medicare coverage in 1997 is 1,500 percent higher than the initial figure. Paul Starr has observed that:

> In setting up Medicare, Congress and the administration were acutely concerned to gain the cooperation of the doctors and hospitals. Consequently, they established buffers between the providers of health care and the federal bureaucracy. Under Part A of Medicare, the law allowed groups of hospitals, extended care facilities, and home health agencies the option of nominating "fiscal intermediaries," instead of dealing directly with the Social Security Administration. These intermediaries were to provide reimbursements, consulting, and auditing services. The federal government was to pay the bills. As expected, the overwhelming majority of hospitals and other institutions nominated Blue Cross. Under Part B, the secretary of HEW [Health, Education, and Welfare] was to choose private insurance agents called "carriers" to serve the same function in a geographical area. The majority of these carriers turned out to be Blue Shield plans. As a result, the administration of Medicare was lodged in the private insurance systems originally established to suit provider interests. And the federal government surrendered direct control of the program and its costs.[6]

More Does Not Mean Better

The erroneous assumption underlying the early decisions about Medicare was that the problem of access to medical care could be solved by pouring dollars into the system, and that no reform of the system itself would be required. After all, we had the best medical care system in the world, didn't we?

The fundamental financing approach enacted under Medicare for both Part A and Part B was "cost reimbursement," which represented an open checkbook if there ever was one. The "cost reimbursement" approach for Part A was eventually widened to include "capital costs," making the Medicare program a major alternative to Hill-Burton, or Hill-Harris, as a source of federal dollars for the expansion and modernization of hospital facilities, including the addition of acute-care beds. As Starr points out:

> The [Medicare] legislation adopted the practice followed by Blue Cross of paying hospitals according to their costs rather than, for example, a schedule of negotiated rates. And in carrying out this provision, the administration agreed to rules for calculating costs that were extremely favorable to the hospital industry. As third parties . . . Medicare and Medicaid reimburse providers on a fee-for-service basis. Since under fee-for-service, doctors and hospitals make more money the more services they provide, they have an incentive to maximize the volume of services. *Third party, fee-for-service payment was the central mechanism of medical inflation.* . . . Medicare and Medicaid, like Blue Cross, chose to reimburse hospitals on the basis of their costs. Under such a system, any institution that reduced its costs would reduce its income, possibly for years to come, since the record of past costs affects future reimbursement levels. On the other hand, the greater its costs, the higher its reimbursements. Thus hospitals were encouraged to solve financing problems, not by minimizing costs but by maximizing reimbursements.[7] (Emphasis added)

Professor Starr observed that the federal agreement to base hospital reimbursement for services to Medicare beneficiaries not merely on the cost of those services, but also on the depreciation of the capital assets of a hospital, its buildings and equipment, opened the way to windfall revenues for hospitals. Starr comments that the depreciation payments provided "the most capital to the hospitals with the newest and most expensive facilities," even though the idea of paying depreciation to a nonprofit institution, i.e., an institution financed by the community, seemed to him "a peculiar idea." This automatic reimbursement from Medicare for capital investments in plant or equipment flowed with no requirements for prioritization, and with no planning or review procedures. As opposed to Hill-Burton, which stipulated such procedures, Medicare offered the hospitals a free ride. Paul Starr points out that these new Medicare policies came at the same time as the sweeping federal health-planning initiatives, which were based on voluntary compliance. Since the newest and most expensively equipped hospitals were now flush with Medicare reimbursements for capital depreciation, their level of voluntary cooperation with community-planning agencies dropped to nil.

Cost reimbursement for hospitals and their fee-for-service physicians has given impetus and credence to the familiar assertion that obtaining a medical license is akin to securing a license to steal.

Variation without Explanation

In his article on variations in hospital use entitled "Which Rate Is Right?" published in the *New England Journal of Medicine,*[8] John Wennberg, M.D., reported on a study by M. R. Chassin and eight colleagues of "Variations in the Use of Medical and Surgical Services by the Medicare population." The researchers found major differences in the rates of utilization of medical and surgical services during calender year 1981, from one area to another, across thirteen large metropolitan areas of the United States. They studied a total of 123 different medical and surgical procedures and found that 67 of these showed *at least threefold variations* between the sites with the highest and lowest rates of use for the specific procedure.

Seventeen years after the 1981 fieldwork, and a dozen years after publication of his article on variations in the rates of utilization of medical resources, Dr. Wennberg is continuing his study of marked variations in the use of surgical and medical services by Medicare beneficiaries. In the 1998 edition of the *Dartmouth Atlas of Health Care in the United States,* published by the American Hospital Publishing Company of Chicago, Wennberg "documents the wide variations in Medicare spending and in the supply of acute care hospital resources and physicians among the nation's hospital referral regions." The atlas goes on to demonstrate that the significant variations in the amount of medical care a person uses "is highly dependent on where they live—on the capacity of the health care system where they live, and on the practice styles of local physicians." Wennberg concludes that, in 1998, "The fundamental questions posed by the *Atlas* are Which rate is right? How much is enough? and What is Fair?" Higher rates of hospitalization continue to occur in those regions with an above average inventory of inpatient beds. No correlation can be found between the *need* for medical care in the population of a specific region, determined by morbidity analyses for each region, and the per capita level of Medicare expenditure in that region. In short, nearly two decades have passed since Dr. Wennberg began the field work that led to the publication of his "Which Rate Is Right" article, and the one thing we can be most certain about is that not much has changed.

Physician free barons are extremely shrewd in the decisions they make that account for these tremendous variations in "practice style." For some medical conditions, like inguinal hernia (a hernia in the groin area), for example, the diagnosis is clear and distinct, and the treatment—surgical repair—is equally so. Dr. Wennberg notes that, in the Chassin study: "inguinal herniorrhaphy shows very little variation between hospital markets or between regions." In other words, the "practice style" of the surgeons across these thirteen regions is not different when it comes to the repair of inguinal hernias. For other medical and surgical procedures that do not present the clear and distinct character of an inguinal hernia, procedures that fall into more of a "gray area" of diagnosis, the variations across the thirteen regions document major differences in "practice style" between and among these same physicians. Consider the conclusions published by Dr. Wennberg:

> Hospital market-area studies provide considerable evidence against the theory that rates of illness explain most of the variation, at least in the use of hospitals. Morbidity surveys have failed to show differences in reported illnesses between populations living in areas with high and low rates of hospital use. More convincing evidence for clinicians, perhaps, is the pattern of variation: The hospitalization rate will bear a close relation to the incidence of an illness only when the related condition is diagnosed with reasonable certainty and when physicians agree on the need to treat the illness in the hospital. Among such conditions are myocardial infarction and hip fractures; admission rates for patients with these conditions are tracers for the incidence of coronary artery disease and fractures and consistently show little variation among hospital markets within a region or state. These conditions are the exception. Admission rates for more than 80 percent of medical conditions, including most orthopedic injuries, such as fractures of the ankle and forearm, and knee and back injuries, and for manifestations of chronic cardiovascular disease other than acute myocardial infarction, such as chest pain, atherosclerosis, and congestive heart failure, are highly variable. For these, the need for hospitalization is less clearly defined and physicians differ from area to area on when hospitalization is appropriate. *The admission rates for these sorts of medical conditions correlate positively with the number of available beds per capita.* Admission rates for hip frac-

ture and myocardial infarction, for example, are approximately equal in Des Moines (5.3 available beds per 1000 population) and Iowa City (3.8 per 1000), whereas the rates for medical conditions with highly variable admission rates, such as hypertension, pneumonia, and atherosclerosis, are twice as high for Medicare enrollees in Des Moines as for those in Iowa City. . . . The rates for most operations, however, are highly variable from one population to another, and the probability of having an operation is conditioned by the supply of surgeons and their opinions on the value of the operation. Whereas in Des Moines and Iowa City the rates of inguinal hernia repair are about the same, the rate of major cardiovascular surgery is twice as high among Medicare enrollees living in Des Moines, even though the incidence of ischemic heart disease is similar, judging from the rates of myocardial infarction. The same pattern is apparent in other states: The incidence of myocardial infarction is about the same in Palo Alto as in North San Diego, but the rate of major cardiovascular surgery is 66 percent higher in North San Diego. . . . [O]utlays from the Medicare program in 1982 were $1,002 in Iowa City . . . while in Des Moines they were 75 percent higher—$1,753 per enrollee. Much of the additional investment in the Des Moines population was for high-variation medical admissions. . . . The study of variations leads naturally to the question, Which rate is right? Physicians and their patients want answers based on the medical model— that is, Which rate makes sense if our goal is to optimize outcome for the patients? For medical conditions associated with highly variable rates of admission, the differences in hospitalization largely reflect different opinions concerning safety. . . . For surgical procedures the outcome question is the efficacy of alternative treatment: When is it appropriate to use one operation instead of another? When is it appropriate to use a medical rather than a surgical approach or simply to watch and wait? Unfortunately , there is little consensus among physicians on questions of safety and efficacy.[9] (Emphasis added)

In the intervening decade since John Wennberg published those words, the advent of Medicare's DRG payment approach has altered the direct correlation between the number of available beds and average length of stay, which should tend to reduce the overall level of hospital utilization in the Medicare program. This is principally because the hospital expects to be paid the DRG, or "diagnosis related group," payment amount for a specific admitting diagnosis, e.g., appendicitis, no matter how long or short a time the patient may occupy a bed, and no matter how much service the patient may receive. There are exceptions made for "outlier" cases, and for complications that may occur during an inpatient stay which, in effect, change the admitting DRG. However, little if any progress has been made in changing the pattern of rates of admission from one hospital region to another, or in the direction of developing a consensus among physician free barons about issues of safety, efficacy, or fairness. The data presented in the previously mentioned 1998 edition of the *Dartmouth Atlas* demonstrate that the question "Which rate is right?" continues to be very pertinent for the future of American medicine. The same data can also be reasonably understood as indicating that the right rate question is being answered by fee-based physicians primarily in terms of their own entrepreneurial self-interest.

The real question becomes: "Which rate will produce the most revenue for my practice?"

The foregoing provides all of the evidence necessary to support the conclusions that (a) the unrestricted production of medical doctors is hazardous to human health; and (b) pouring dollars into the healthcare system in the absence of a major reconstruction of the American medical guild's current scheme of ideas can only worsen the present crisis, thereby accelerating the date of eventual national bankruptcy.

The University of Pennsylvania School of Medicine was established in 1765, followed by the Columbia University College of Physicians and Surgeons in 1767, by Harvard Medical School in 1782, and by Dartmouth Medical School in 1797. America entered the nineteenth century with four university-based factories for the production of medical doctors. All of them were private institutions. Twenty-seven university medical schools, all of which continue in existence today, were established during the first half of the nineteenth century, bringing the total to thirty-one. Fourteen of these new schools were public institutions. Starting with the watershed year of 1859, in which Darwin published his *Origin of Species,* and during the next century, fifty-six more university-based medical schools opened their doors to medical students, raising the total to eighty-seven. Thirty-three of these were public facilities, and all fifty-six schools remain in operation today as fully accredited institutions.

During the 195 years from 1765 through 1959, therefore, American society had supported the creation of eighty-seven university-based physician-production facilities. During the eighteen-year period from 1960 to 1978, the U.S. Congress provided financing for medical school construction and medical education resulting in a 44 percent increase in the number of university-based physician-production facilities, with the addition of thirty-eight new fully accredited institutions, bringing the total to 125. Twenty-nine of these new schools, or 76 percent of them, were public institutions. During these eighteen years, new medical schools were created at a rate fifty-two times the growth rate for medical schools during the previous two centuries. These numbers take into account only fully accredited medical schools in the United States. There are a number of other medical schools operating in the country which have not attained full accreditation from the Liaison Committee on Medical Education (LCME).

It is eminently reasonable and justifiable to state that, had Congress not acted with such folly in stimulating this outlandish increase in physician-production facilities during those eighteen years, the nation would not be facing the crises in medical care that threaten it today: neither the crisis of radical escalation in expenditures nor the crisis in worsening morbidity and mortality statistics. These crises can each be traced directly to the radical oversupply of practicing physicians in the United States today, an oversupply that continues to escalate.

In an unusual stroke of sheer good fortune for the American public, no additional medical schools with full LCME accreditation have been brought on line since 1978.

The annual financial review of all 125 accredited medical schools is administered by the LCME. Based upon the latest report of this annual review, published in the September 4, 1996 issue of *JAMA*, federal and state subsidies for these schools, including direct federal GME (Graduate Medical Education) payments, research grants and contracts, totaled $8.4 billion for fiscal year 1995. In addition, the Congressional Budget Office (CBO) reported in May of 1996 that the Medicare program paid an additional $4.5 billion in fiscal year 1995 in "indirect medical education" (IME) adjustments "for its share of the costs of teaching activities related to patient care at teaching hospitals." These public GME expenditures of $12.9 billion for fiscal year 1995 constituted 44 percent of the total revenues for these 125 medical schools. Not included in the reports of this astonishing level of continuing governmental subsidy of medical education is a breakdown of the federal and state revenues received by medical school faculty for "medical services" provided to Medicare and Medicaid beneficiaries in the university hospitals and clinics affiliated with these medical schools.

The conclusion to the *JAMA* report on LCME's annual financial review of the 125 accredited medical schools includes the following statements:

> Medical education is supported by tuition, which continues to increase. For public schools, however, a more significant source of support for this activity is state and local government appropriations, which have not generally kept pace with inflation. . . . Federal research funding continues to increase, but at a slower rate than in former decades. Also, more recent restrictions on the reimbursement of F&A (facilities & administrative) costs have diminished schools' ability to recover the costs of essential infrastructure requirements. . . . Although revenues continue to grow, a careful review of the data reveals an increased stress on the ability of medical schools to accomplish their academic mission.[10]

In the light of what has been demonstrated about the perverse relationships which exist between the ratio of surgeons to population on the one hand, and the incidence of unnecessary surgeries on the other; or between the ratio of acute-care hospital beds to population and the higher level of infant mortality among the women with the greater access to those beds, two questions about these ongoing subsidies cry out for answers:

(a) How is it possible for elected officials to morally justify an annual expenditure of $12.9 billion in federal and state taxpayer funds to subsidize the production of medical doctors who are already in radical oversupply, an excess of physicians that is resulting in medically unnecessary procedures being performed on a scale that is worsening the health status of the American people?

(b) How is it possible for elected officials to justify in terms of basic fiscal responsibility an annual subsidy of $12.9 billion in federal and state monies, an expenditure that can only worsen a physician oversupply already so large that it is threatening to cripple the national economy?

If the U.S. Congress is seriously interested in controlling expenditures for such entitlement programs as Medicare and Medicaid, and is serious about controlling healthcare expenditures generally, then taking strong action to curtail and contain the *supply* of physicians would constitute the most rational and logical first step. Instead, the persistent and destructive subsidizing of medical schools and medical research continues, during a time when these excessive capacities should be reduced by at least one-half.

The Graduate Medical Education National Advisory Committee (GMENAC) was chartered by the federal government for the period of April 20, 1976, through September 30, 1980. The purpose of the committee was "to analyze the distribution among specialties of physicians and residents and to evaluate alternative approaches to ensure an appropriate balance . . . and make recommendations to the Secretary (of Health, Education, and Welfare) on overall strategies on the present and future supply and requirements of physicians by specialty . . . (and) translation of physician requirements into a range of types and numbers of graduate training opportunities needed to approach a more desirable distribution of physician services." At the termination of its service, the committee consisted of twenty-two members, fifteen of them being physicians.

Writing on this subject in 1985, Eli Ginzberg, a professor of economics and director of the Eisenhower Center for the Conservation of Human Resources at Columbia University made the following observation:

> The leadership of the medical community has opposed many of the federal initiatives that have been identified and has not supported the GMENAC report submitted to the Secretary of HEW in 1980, which warned of the urgent need for corrective action to prevent the large surplus of physicians that will otherwise be manifest by 1990 and the even larger surplus by 2000. . . . As we look at the plethora of organized medical groups, from county medical societies to residency review committees, it is difficult to identify their principal objectives and goals other than a continuing emphasis on noninterference with patient-physician relationships, concern with the rise of malpractice litigation but little success in stemming it, and broad support for specialization and high-tech medical care.[11]

The American medical guild paid no attention to the report by GMENAC, and neither did Congress. The "urgent need for corrective action" was ignored, and, in the absence of any action, the nation is currently reaping the predicted whirlwind.

These days, members of Congress increasingly talk about market forces as the source of solution for persistent social problems. The Majority Leader of the House of Representatives, Dick Armey, put it this way: "The market is rational and the government is dumb." (This is the first on a list of "Armey's Axioms" published on the Majority leader's personal website called Dick Armey's Reading Room.) In the case of medicine, however, as has been noted, market forces as currently manifest can only worsen the situation, for the clear and simple reason that the *supplier* is the chief regulator of *demand.* The more suppliers, the higher the level of demand. In testimony before the Senate Finance Committee's Health Subcommittee eighteen years ago, Bert Seidman of the AFL-CIO's Department of Social Security, speaking in opposition to a catastrophic health-insurance bill (S.350), and to a companion bill called the Medical Assistance Reform Act of 1979 (S.351), said the following:

> Mr. Chairman, what is conspicuously absent from both bills is a rudimentary understanding of the basic economics of the health care industry. The laws of supply and demand are skewed beyond recognition in this industry. Doctors—not patients—control the demand for medical services. It is the doctor who decides whether a patient goes to a hospital or receives much less expensive treatment on an outpatient basis. It is the doctor who decides when a patient can be transferred to an extended care facility. It is the doctor who decides when the patient can be discharged from a hospital or nursing home. It is the doctor who decides how often the patient should come to the office for treatment, and the number of hospital visits that need to be made by the doctor. It is the doctor who decides what laboratory tests or diagnostic procedures need to be performed. It is the doctor who prescribes drugs, either by brand name or less costly but equally effective generic equivalents. It is the patient's physician who leaves instructions with the house staff or the nurse. Patients know this. When patients go to a physician with symptoms—perhaps for a physical examination—they place themselves under the doctor's direction.[12]

Despite the recent success the AMA has had in convincing many people of the falsehood that HMOs and "managed-care" plans, through their administrative employees, control medical decisions affecting their members, with the result that doctors are no longer the sole regulators of the demand for medical services, these are in fact the economic forces that remain at work in the medical-care marketplace today. Given these forces, and recognizing that the Congress has been effectively persuaded by the medical guild to do nothing that could possibly alter those forces, there is at present no discernable limit to how high expenditures for medical care may go. The GMENAC projections of a "worst case" increase in the oversupply of physicians have already been surpassed and, under the scheme of ideas adopted by the free barons of American medicine, the progression toward national bankruptcy is speeding up. Patients are not alone in "placing themselves under the doctor's direction," for Congress has persistently done exactly the same thing. The Congress has steadfastly aligned itself with George Bernard Shaw's dictum that: "We have not lost faith, but we have transferred it from God to the medical profession."

Graduating a physician from an accredited medical school represents a commitment by the American people to an annuity of $150,000 (AMA's current claim of median annual physician income) for a period of forty years—a promise to pay $6 million per physician. (There are, it should be noted, cardiovascular surgeons today who produce that much income—$6 million—in the space of two years). However, the median annual physician income of $150,000 must be multiplied by ten to obtain the real cost to society of each graduating physician, since the total outlays for medical care equate to over ten times the aggregate median net income (of $150,000) for all active physicians; and since the licensed physician is the only actor within the medical cosmos with the authority to generate expenditure. Total annual health expenditures of $1 trillion divided by 600,000 active physicians equals $1,666,666 in average annual expenditure per active physician. (Contrary to the self-serving disinformation that the AMA has been effectively marketing to the American public, HMOs and "managed-care" health plans have no direct role in generating or depressing expenditures for medical care. The only role that health plans can legally and appropriately play is a *benefit interpretation* role, i.e., whether a procedure or treatment the physician recommends is covered by the contract that the member signed, or not. No medical decisions are involved here, only decisions about who is responsible for payment. Physicians who believe that their recommended treatment is medically necessary for the patient ought to provide the care forthwith, and let payment issues be settled after the patient has been restored to health.) Thus the true annuity undertaken by society for each graduating physician today is not $150,000 but nearly $1.7 million—adding up over forty years to a staggering promise-to-pay averaging $66 million per physician. And this is using 1996 prices.

If it is accurate to state, as I believe, that there are currently twice as many practicing physicians in the United States as would be optimal; and if society's annuity for each of these doctors is as calculated above; then Americans can anticipate having to come up with $18 trillion over the next forty years to subsidize the physician oversupply that exists *today*, an excess of at least 225,000 practicing physicians. The ten-year cost of subsidizing this oversupply will be $4.5 trillion; and the five-year cost—that is, between 1997 and 2002—will be $2.25 trillion, the equivalent of *two and a quarter years of total national health care expenditures* at the current level of outlay.

In view of the fact that the Congress and the states are continuing to support nearly one-third of the cost of producing more than 16,000 new physicians each year, counting only the U.S. graduates of LCME-accredited programs, the current oversupply is bound to increase. The Pew Health Professions Commission reported an excess of 90 physicians per 100,000 population in 1995, and projected that this would increase by 55 percent, to an excess of 140 per 100,000, by the turn of the century.[13] As this oversupply continues to increase, so will the unconscionable and unsupportable financial burden on American society. How is it possible for elected officials, ostensibly committed to carrying on the public business, to justify the continuation of these massive physician-production subsidies, from either a moral or an economic point of view? The answer is, of course, that it is *not* possible.

Aside from the issue of the continuous production of a ravaging oversupply of physicians, America's medical schools are fully engaged in the commission of other grievous sins against society. In a discussion of the explosion of medical specialization in chapter 3, reference is made to the long and growing list of distinct "specialties." A 1996 report of resident physicians in accredited "specialty" graduate programs in the United States lists a total of eighty-seven different "specialty" and "subspecialty" residencies available to qualified medical school graduates. Ninety-one percent of these graduates do go on to a residency program, and the number of "specialties" is now almost four and a half times what it was in America before Darwin. Not more than a handful of these eighty-seven "specialty" and "subspecialty" residencies involve additional training in primary care: family practice, general pediatrics, internal medicine, and some aspects of obstetrics.

The free barons who are the professors of medicine in the 125 LCME-accredited medical schools in the United States share a general attitude of contempt for primary care as a field of medical practice. Few if any of them would consider a career in primary care for themselves, and they therefore consider anyone who would do so as being beneath them. Any medical student or resident who is interested in primary care, and who strikes one of these professors as bright and competent, is almost certainly going to hear the following advice: *"You are far too intelligent to spend your life in primary care. You should consider a residency in radiology (or one of the 80-odd other options). You will earn three or four times as much money, and work half the hours. Take my advice, switch from primary care before it is too late."*

A Chill Where Warmth Is Needed

In a descriptive study published in *JAMA* in 1996, a Harvard Medical School physician and three Ph.D.s affiliated with Harvard University presented their findings regarding academia's attitudes toward primary care. The "comment" section of the study included the following statements:

> This study presents a panoramic representation of the climate for primary care in AHCs (academic health centers). The use of a national probability sample enables us to generalize to the universe of medical students, residents, faculty, and academic leaders. Our data demonstrate that, in spite of secular changes in the health care system and in medical education, the environment within AHCs is chilly for primary care education and practice. We show that the composition of the faculty and the culture, values and educational practices of large segments of the academic medical community and system are poorly aligned with the goals of enhancing the education and environment for primary care. The multiple perspectives offered in this study and the convergence of opinion among so many different constituents of the AHCs indicate that the chilly climate is a pervasive phenomenon. . . . Our data showing that even primary care-oriented faculty and learners demonstrate negative attitudes about their own (collective) competence suggest that the chilly climate for primary care adversely influ-

ences primary care faculty and learners. The experience of being immersed in an academic culture that values specialty practice and devalues generalism may compromise enthusiasm for primary care education and practice. While a case might be made for specialty care of more serious medical problems, the fact that 30% of the clinical faculty do not see generalists as the physicians best suited to provide care for less serious illnesses raises questions about what role they do perceive for generalists in the health care system. The near universality of the perception that academically capable students are not encouraged toward primary care is another indicator of the low regard for generalism in the academic medicine community. . . . [T]he values of traditional biomedicine and medical education continue to emphasize specialized knowledge and competence as opposed to breadth of knowledge; biological factors as opposed to social and emotional factors in health; and inpatient as opposed to outpatient care and training. . . . While interprofessional rivalries and stereotypes are an inevitable feature of academic medicine, we believe that the negativity toward primary care goes beyond benign professional rivalry and is deeply rooted in the culture of medicine. The presence of a chilly climate for primary care in AHCs represents a barrier to primary care career choice and education and compromises the quality of professional life for primary care-oriented students, residents, and faculty. Major changes in the culture of AHCs will be necessary to make their climate hospitable for primary care. . . . If medical educators seek to optimize enthusiasm and preparation for primary care careers, they must develop approaches to changing the attitudes, values, and composition of their faculties.[14]

Readers would be well advised not to hold your breath while awaiting these changes.

Twenty years ago, the Health Professions Educational Assistance Act of 1976 declared that "there is no longer a shortage of physicians but rather a maldistribution of physicians, both geographically and by specialty." Twenty-five years ago, the Study of Surgical Services in the United States (SOSSUS) reported "an excess number of surgeons being certified in surgery, neurosurgery, ophthalmology, orthopedics, obstetrics-gynecology, thoracic surgery, and plastic surgery."[15] Twenty years ago, in an article in the *Journal of Medical Education* entitled "U.S. Health Manpower Policy: Will the Benefits Justify the Costs?" J. H. Morrow and A. B. Edwards recommended that:

first-year residency positions be reduced in most specialties, including pediatrics, dermatology, neurology, pathology, and radiology in addition to most of the surgical specialties; substantial increases in first year residency positions . . . (are) . . . recommended in only one field—family practice.[16]

The recommendations by Morrow and Edwards, particularly with regard to the surgical specialties, were identical to those made in the SOSSUS study cited above. In a 1981 article in the *New England Journal of Medicine*, D. C. Williams reported on his followup of the SOSSUS study in the state of Rhode Island. Dr. Williams concluded:

> As of 1977, the SOSSUS recommendations [to limit the number of physicians performing operations and reduce the number of surgeons being trained] were having no demonstrable impact in Rhode Island. The number of surgeons was continuing to increase without apparent need, as judged by operative workloads.[17]

The Congress has turned a deaf ear to all of these cogent and crucial warnings.

In his preface to *Science and the Modern World*, Alfred North Whitehead wrote: "The present book embodies a study of some aspects of Western culture during the past three centuries, in so far as it has been influenced by the development of science." The book consisted of his Lowell Lectures, which were delivered in 1925. It is in these lectures that Whitehead identifies and delineates the *Fallacy of Misplaced Concreteness* (referenced in chapter 3), as being ingredient in the foundations of the scientific scheme of the seventeenth century. It is this very fallacy of thinking, more than any single factor other than human greed, which accounts for the misdirections and misadventures characteristic of contemporary American medicine, including the now well-documented fact that a "chilly" climate exists in academic medicine toward family practice and toward the few other medical disciplines that fall under the definition of primary care.

The concreteness which Whitehead has termed "misplaced" stems principally from the mistaking of "our abstractions for concrete realities."[18] The point has been made that the scheme of ideas which overarches the theory and practice of contemporary American medicine is rooted in the "famous mechanistic theory of nature."[19] For example, the concept of a "living body" is an abstraction within medical epistemology that is consistently mistaken for the concrete reality, which, in fact, is an organism with a specific genetic and environmental history, having complex and ongoing biochemical, physiological, and psychological processes. The current method of disease classification in American medicine—a system of abstractions—is a clear example of *misplaced concreteness,* in that its taproot springs from mistaking the abstraction "living body" for the concrete reality "organism with a specific genetic and environmental history, having complex and ongoing biochemical, physiological, and psychological processes." This is certainly not to argue that medicine needs to abandon its abstractions—quite the contrary. Ian R. McWhinney, M.D., who is professor emeritus of the Department of Family Medicine at the University of Western Ontario, and who is the cofounder of the Centre for Studies in Family Medicine at the University, has made these observations:

> Abstraction is an essential part of the scientific method, but its danger is that we can so easily become the prisoners of our abstractions. "The disadvantage of exclusive attention to a group of abstractions," wrote Whitehead, "however well founded, is that, by the nature of the case, you have abstracted from the remainder of things. Insofar as the excluded things are important in your experience, your modes of thought are not fitted to deal with them. You cannot think without abstractions: accordingly, it is of the utmost importance to be vigilant in critically revising your modes of abstraction. . . . A civilization which cannot burst through its current abstractions is doomed to sterility after a very limited period of progress."[20]

Over the ages, medicine has been defined as both a science and an art. One of the reasons that American medicine is more the latter than the former is the fact that physician free barons rarely if ever examine or rethink their own basic assumptions, their scheme of ideas, or their abstractions. The way in which diabetes mellitus is generally being treated in the United States today provides an excellent illustration of the fallacy of misplaced concreteness at work: the attention given to the abstractions "living body," "organ," and "pancreas" leads the physician to "abstract from the remainder of things. Insofar as the excluded things are important . . . your modes of thought are not fitted to deal with them."[21] (See chapter 5, pages 205–14 for a review of diabetes care in America, including a comparison of recently reported population-based mortality outcomes of diabetes in the United States and the United Kingdom). It is an irreducible fact that the health care system in the United States today "lacks a . . . delivery system appropriate for the needs of people with diabetes."[22] One reason for the well-documented inadequacy of diabetes care is *misplaced concreteness*: to the extent that physicians cannot "burst through" their conventional abstractions, no progress in terms of *science* is possible.

So-called modern medicine persistently presents examples of this fallacy of misplaced concreteness, occurring throughout the length and breadth of even its most celebrated clinical performances. Within the scheme of ideas that the American medical guild has adopted, the "remainder of things" is continuously being left out of the processes of clinical observation and judgment. To quote Whitehead on the fate of a system "which cannot burst through its current abstractions," medicine in the United States is thereby "doomed to sterility after a very limited period of progress." The only way out of this box in which "the best medical system in the world" currently finds itself will be a thoroughgoing reconstruction of the current scheme of ideas, of contemporary medical epistemology, and of academic medicine. Unfortunately, the physician free barons of America, by their nature and essence, will be disinclined to undertake the necessary reconstructions.

Family medicine, as a science and as an art, holds out the best chance for American medicine to overcome the intellectual ravages caused by the fallacy of *misplaced concreteness,* and by academic medicine's bifurcation of "basic science" and "clinical medicine" on the one hand, and its confusion of science and technology on the other hand. In his article "Family Medicine as a Science," Professor McWhinney states:

> It is in its attitude to accurate observation—what Whitehead called "brute fact"—that scientific thought differs from medieval thought. Medieval thinkers were intensely rational, but their arguments were based on *a priori* assumptions rather than verified facts of experience. A devotion to facts, however, is not in itself sufficient to define the scientific method. The other essential activity of science is the formulation of explanatory theories which can be tested against experience. It is theory which organizes and gives meaning to our data, helps us to formulate problems, and provides the basis

for the interpretation of empirical findings. . . . One cannot observe without having some theory about the objects to be observed. The theory may
not be an original one; it may not even be consciously held; it will never-
theless be a world view, derived from our culture and formal education,
about how phenomena are to be classified and valued. . . . The objects of
science, then, are intellectual constructs. In medicine, the "diseases" which
we describe have no real existence; they are abstractions which we invent
to bring order to a mass of data about illness. . . . So far, family medicine
seems to have accepted without question medicine's current system of
abstractions, i.e., its method of classifying diseases. We have done this even
though it often fits poorly with the "brute facts" of general practice. We
continue, for example, to perform morbidity surveys in which we accept
without question concepts like "psychiatric illness." And we continue to
find it very difficult to obtain results which are consistent from one physician to another. . . . Perhaps we are on the brink of a change of paradigm in
medicine. If we are, then I suggest that it is more likely to come from
family medicine than any other field, because it is in family medicine that
we see most clearly the incongruities of our current system of abstractions.

We have become accustomed in medicine to distinguishing between basic
science and clinical medicine. These terms are not often defined but I often
suspect that the term "basic" is used to imply that chemistry, physics,
physiology, anatomy, and pharmacology are more scientific and fundamental than clinical medicine. *This is really the opposite of the truth* (emphasis
mine), for it would be impossible to apply advances in basic science
without a body of scientific knowledge which is only obtainable from clinical observation. In the study of human illness, the ultimate test of any
chemical or physical analysis must be: what are its implications for the survival and functioning of the whole organism? And this is a question which
can only be answered by clinical observation. . . . Clinical observation,
then, is not only a scientific discipline, but it is *the* science of medicine. . . .
Clinical medicine, like astronomy, ethology, anthropology, and a large part
of biology, is an observational science. It is one of those sciences which, in
[John] Ryle's words, tries to "establish the truth of things by observing and
recording, by classification and analysis." We must go on to acknowledge,
however, that clinical observation has been a much neglected science in our
own time. In his book, *Clinical Judgment,* Feinstein has commented: "Medical taxonomy has given . . . (the clinician) classifications for the host and
for the disease, but not for the illness of the patient who is the diseased

host. Lacking any formal means of classifying clinical observations, the clinician has no place to put the information when he communicates with himself or with his colleagues."[23]

It would be difficult to come by a more perfect illustration of the fallacy of misplaced concreteness than this: in the contemporary medical classification system, the abstractions "disease" and "host" have been systematically put in the place of the concrete reality—the patient—and the clinician is left without a place to record his clinical observations of the only concrete reality before him. Since clinical observation "is *the* science of medicine," and since the prevailing scheme of ideas deprives the clinician of a means of classifying observations of the nonabstract, concretely real patient, it is clear that contemporary clinical medicine in the United States cannot qualify as a science. Instead, contemporary medicine is fundamentally *technology* being marketed and misperceived as science. Ian McWhinney comments on this point as follows:

Although medicine can be described as an observational science, most of medical knowledge would be more correctly classified as technological rather than scientific. . . . It is true that science and technology have in modern times become so interwoven that it is difficult to tell them apart. . . . One might be forgiven for thinking that there is no longer any useful distinction between them; scientists use tools, and scientific research itself is a technical and a craft skill; technologists make precise observations and develop theories which can make an important contribution to our understanding. Moreover, the methods which technologists use for evaluating their tools are the same as those which scientists use for testing their hypotheses. . . . There are also, however, some important differences. . . . A scientific discovery deepens our understanding of nature; a technological invention, in [Michael] Polanyi's words, "establishes a new operational principle serving some acknowledged advantage." The test of a scientific discovery is the question, Is it true? The test of a technological invention is the question, Does it work? A scientific discovery can be superseded only by another discovery which brings us nearer to the truth. A technological invention can be superseded by another invention, or by a change in the way a process or its outcomes are valued by society.[24]

The physician free barons of the American medical guild have flourished during the period since Flexner's report primarily on the basis of having effectively misrepresented technological invention as scientific discovery. Barry Marshall, M.D., deserves credit for a major scientific discovery, the *helicobacter* bacterium as the cause of most stomach ulcers. The free barons and the top guns of the American guild, some of whose technological tools and ulcer surgery practices were doomed to obsolescence by Marshall's scientific discovery, fought him to a standstill for ten years, until the "brute facts" of clinical observation finally prevailed.

Given the reception accorded Barry Marshall when he first informed his medical colleagues of his scientific discovery, which can generously be characterized as mocking disbelief, it is no stretch from there to the conclusion that what is today termed "basic science" by academic medicine is much more at the service of promoting technological invention than supporting true scientific discovery. The prevailing scheme of ideas and the erroneous epistemology of contemporary medicine make this conclusion inevitable.

Writing on "The Nature of Medical Knowledge," McWhinney has observed the following:

> One of the greatest objections to the idea of the family doctor has been that one physician cannot effectively master the science of medicine. The root of this objection is a concept of medical knowledge that I hold to be fallacious. I call it "the lump fallacy." According to this view, knowledge is a lump of material that grows by accretion. Having reached a certain size, it becomes too large to be assimilated and must be broken up into smaller lumps. These smaller lumps, however, continue to grow at an ever increasing rate and in their turn have to be fragmented, and so on. This view of knowledge is surely a distortion of the truth. A physician uses three kinds of knowledge. The first, which I will call information, is the only one to which the simile of a material mass ran be applied; the second, clinical craftsmanship, is a skill; the third, which I will call insight and awareness, is an integral part of the personality. These three kinds of knowledge are acquired in quite different ways. Information comes from observation, listening, and reading; clinical skill, like other skills, comes from constant practice and the emulation of others; insight and awareness come from human intercourse and deep reflection on the self and on experience. Excellence in one of these areas of knowledge does not in any way guarantee excellence in the others. One tends to think of poor physicians as badly informed physicians. But everyone has encountered superbly informed

physicians who can quote all the latest references, but are woefully lacking in clinical judgment, and also excellent clinicians who in their dealings with people are incredibly naive. Excellence in medicine requires a blend of all kinds of knowledge. My own observation is that error in medicine arises more from a failure of skill or insight than from a lack of information. A lack of information is most readily remedied by reference to book or consultant. Defects of skill or insight are far more difficult to remedy— not least because the physician, lacking self-knowledge, cannot recognize his own failings. It is apparent, therefore, why I consider the conventional view of medical knowledge to be a very limited one. . . . It is also apparent why I do not believe that a family doctor need sacrifice any of this vital type of knowledge. On the contrary, by caring for the whole family, he stands to gain personal knowledge that can be gained in no other way.[25]

With its prevailing theory of knowledge so fundamentally flawed, and given the fact that the Congress listens only to the "leaders" of academic medicine in deciding on massive investments in medical education and research, can it be any wonder that federal expenditures for medical research are misdirected and wrongheaded? If family medicine provides the fundamental laboratory for carrying on *the* science of medicine; and if academic medicine irrefutably exhibits a fundamental disrespect and a "chilly climate" for family medicine, and for primary care in general (rooted in academia's ignorance of the role and value of the generalist in scientific discovery); then the brute fact that must be faced is that the academic context into which federal outlays for medical research are now being heavily invested constitutes a virtual guarantee that the only legitimate ends that legislators could possibly have for making these huge investments of taxpayer dollars cannot and will not be realized.

The erroneous assumptions by Congress at work in this instance are: (a) that the distinctions between scientific discovery and technological invention are unimportant; and, (b) that academic medicine's bifurcation of "basic science" and "clinical medicine" can be not only tolerated, but handsomely supported. This is gargantuan folly.

The Congressional Record

Between 1963 and 1988, the Congress enacted dozens of laws aimed at improving medical care in the United States. The Health Professions Educational Assistance Act of 1963 provided construction and renovation grants to medical schools, as well as financial aid to medical students. These federal efforts to increase manpower resulted in a 50 percent increase in the number of practicing physicians within a decade. There were over 375,000 active physicians on line by 1976, up from 250,000 in the early 1960s. Many other laws, commonly identified by their acronyms, constituted an alphabet soup of legislative initiatives that have reflected conflicting and often contradictory purposes, e.g., the purpose of insuring adequate regulatory control over federally funded programs was inevitably conditioned by the felt need to accommodate the concerns and interests of the medical guild, as well as the interests of those sponsoring the guild's professional workshops—the hospitals. Recognition of the failure to achieve the former purpose due to the conflicting desire to fulfill the latter "felt need" led the Congress to belatedly enact a series of laws intended to cure the galloping epidemic of radical inflation in medical and hospital-care expenditures which had resulted from that failure. Harvard sociologist Paul Starr has made the following observations:

> The same Congress that enacted Medicare adopted . . . the Regional Medical Programs (RMPs) [which] . . . is particularly revealing of the tilt toward the hospitals and medical schools that persisted in government policy even as it became more redistributive in its objectives. In 1964 a Presidential Commission on Heart Disease, Cancer and Stroke (the Debakey Commission) . . . recommended a massive commitment of federal funds to establish "a national network of regional centers, local diagnostic and treatment stations, and medical complexes designed to unite the worlds of scientific research, medical education, and medical care." The report paid no attention to any environmental, nutritional, or other public health and preventive concerns. Like the report of the Hospital Commission of the 1940s, the Debakey Commission report was a classic of the kind of myopia that the medical establishment of the mid-twentieth century confused with visionary ideals. . . . The aim was to make medical services more available, but there was little thought as to whether such an investment might actually make any difference in health.[26]

After RMPs came PSROs (Professional Standards Review Organization), proposed by the AMA in response to the Nixon administration's "program review teams," initially intended to control Medicare expenditures by giving the power to deny payment for Medicare services that the review body, including nonphysician consumer representatives, deemed to be unnecessary. This Nixon initiative in 1970 was killed by the AMA lobby, and in 1972, the PSRO legislation was passed, with changes made to accommodate all AMA objections. The review bodies would be made up of physicians only, and they would not have the power to deny payment. At the time, consumer advocate Ralph Nader's group aptly described the new PSRO law as "assigning the fox to guard the henhouse." At federal expense, physician committees were established throughout the nation with the principal goal of curbing unnecessary hospital use within the prevailing cost-reimbursement environment.

As noted earlier, Nixon's announcement of a "new national health strategy" centered on federal grants and loans to create HMOs, including a mandate for employers of twenty-five or more to offer the federally "qualified" plans to their employees, was viewed by the medical guild as an act of treason. In his book *The Social Transformation of American Medicine,* Paul Starr made the following observations:

> In August of 1971, President Nixon imposed a general wage-price freeze. When modified that December, the program singled medical care out for special treatment, limiting doctor's fees to annual increases of 2.5 percent and hospital charges to increases of 6 percent (about half the inflation rate in medical care preceding the freeze). And when price controls were lifted in January, 1973, they were retained only for health care and for the food, oil and construction industries. The decision to maintain controls on health care reflected concern about the structural flaws in the industry that were felt likely to generate raging inflation again. Once more, a specific interest of the state was involved: Health expenditures had risen from 4.4 percent of the federal budget in 1965 to 11.3 percent in 1973.[27]

Why, during the early 1970s, would Richard M. Nixon take such aggressive actions in contravention of the interests and wishes of the American medical guild? In January of 1970, *Fortune* magazine published a special edition on medical care that revealed the climate of opinion prevailing at the time. The *Fortune* publication included the finding that medical care in America was

> on the brink of chaos. . . . Much of U.S. medical care, particularly the everyday business of preventing and treating routine illnesses, is inferior in quality, wastefully dispensed, and inequitably financed. Medical manpower and facilities are so maldistributed that large segments of the population, especially the urban poor and those in rural areas, get virtually no care at all—even though their illnesses are most numerous and, in a medical sense, often easy to cure. Whether poor or not, most Americans are badly served by the obsolete, over-strained medical system that has grown up around them helter-skelter. . . . The time has come for radical change.[28]

This was not the "liberal press" that Nixon scorned, but *Fortune* magazine.

Despite this tangible climate of opinion, however, there was one glaring and major exemption apparent in the Nixon administration's efforts to "get tough" with the American medical guild and its hospital workshops. Sociologist Paul Starr pointed out this flaw as follows:

> The least controversial part of Nixon's 1971 national health "strategy" was a call to increase the supply of physicians and change the method of subsidizing medical schools. The administration was much influenced by a report of the Carnegie Commission on Higher Education, which urged that more support to medical schools be given in the form of "capitation grants" (so many dollars per student) with bonuses for increased enrollment. In 1971 Congress introduced the capitation grants in a revised Health Manpower Act.[29]

It is noteworthy that Abraham Flexner's 1910 report on the reconstruction of American medical education was funded by the Carnegie Foundation.

Following Nixon's resignation, in 1974 Gerald Ford asked the Congress to enact a national health-insurance program. Fifteen months later he pulled back, saying it would only worsen the inflation of healthcare costs. His secretary of the treasury, William Simon, was quoted at the time as saying that national health insurance "would be an unmitigated disaster that could bankrupt the country."[30] Bill Simon was absolutely correct.

As early as 1966, the Congress passed Comprehensive Health Planning

(CHP) legislation to stimulate more rational and sensible planning of investments in the construction or expansion of hospitals and other diagnostic and
treatment facilities. However, as noted author and social scientist Paul Starr
has observed, "[T]he whole effort was vitiated from the start by the refusal to
give the agencies any control over the allocation of health care capital or the
reimbursement system that determined the flow of revenues."[31] The rapid
increases in healthcare spending, and the major impact these radically
increased expenditures were having on the federal treasury, eventually led the
Congress to take action. Eighteen years after its enactment of CHP, in 1974,
Congress passed the National Health Planning and Resource Development
Act, designed to create a new system of planning in health care. The new law
created and funded Health Systems Agencies (HSAs) throughout the
country. These agencies were:

> run by boards with consumer majorities representative of their areas. But
> the HSAs were not given any decision-making power; they were to draw
> up three-year Health System Plans, review proposals for new projects, and
> send recommendations to the states on certificates of need and to Wash-
> ington on proposed uses of certain federal funds. All states were required
> to pass certificate-of-need legislation and to establish State Health Plan-
> ning and Development Agencies (SHPDAs) and Statewide Health Coordi-
> nating Councils (SHCCs). . . . The law seemed to be a decisive rejection of
> the view that the market could correct itself and that the doctors and hos-
> pitals had the last word on how medical care ought to be organized. The
> AMA saw the law the same way. Russell Roth, an AMA president, com-
> plained that doctors and administrators had been "pointedly relegated to a
> minor role" and spoke of "the general resentment in the professional com-
> munity" that it wasn't entrusted with leadership of the effort. Of the con-
> sumers' role, Roth observed, "Passengers who insist on flying the aircraft
> are called hijackers!"[32]

In using this simile, Dr. Roth conveniently overlooked the basic economic fact that the "hijackers" he refers to were paying the salaries of the
"pilots." In any event, the consumer-driven HSAs did not produce a breakthrough in health planning. Our history indicates that the frontier experience undoubtedly contributed many positive and enduring strengths to
American culture, however, an affection for orderly planning was not one of

them. The history of the now-defunct federally supported planning bodies confirms this cultural predilection. There is some evidence that construction of hospitals and other healthcare facilities was dampened slightly, on a nationwide basis, by the HSAs; and to a more significant degree within a handful of states where strong regional planning efforts did in fact succeed. However, the overall planning effort that the 93rd Congress saw fit to stimulate and to finance has largely amounted to a waste of time, effort, and treasure. In addition, the planning structures that evolved under the HSA legislation created such elaborate bureaucratic mazes as to present a perfect target for physician free barons, hospital administrators and their lobbyists, in their very successful and persistent efforts to attack "big government" solutions, and to propagate the gospel of market competition, free of governmental regulation or interference, as the only way to resolve the "crisis" in medical care.

In its disappointment over the predictable signs that PSROs were not helping in any significant degree, Congress turned to the Prospective Payment System (PPS)—probably the one and only federal healthcare legislative initiative of the past thirty-five years that can be judged intelligent. This legislation brought a gradual end to the cost-based reimbursement of hospitals by the Medicare program. The new payment approach was based upon the delineation of DRGs (diagnostic related groups) for which a defined payment was established for each area, regardless of the specific services provided to an individual patient admitted under a given DRG code. It took several years to work the bugs out of this system, and many hospitals figured out ways to improve their profits during these initial years under DRG payments. A 1987 article in the *Washington Post* reported that:

> Hospitals made profits averaging 12 to 15 percent on Medicare patients in 1984 and 1985, far higher than before Medicare's new cost-control payment system began a year earlier, three government agencies told Congress. "Is this a reasonable average margin?" House Ways and Means health subcommittee Chairman Fortney H. (Pete) Stark (D. Calif.) asked incredulously. . . . Before the system began in 1983, a "3 percent hospital profit margin" was "historically allowed by Medicare," said Caroll L. Estes. . . . Many at the hearing said the profit margins appear so large that there will be moves to block a substantial increase in government payment rates to hospitals in fiscal 1988.[33]

Although hospital profits from the Medicare line of business went up smartly under DRG payment, for the first time in the century it was not because costs had been padded at the urging of hospital administrators. In the pre-DRG mode department supervisors were given revenue targets to meet. If the laundry department revenues were low, it was no trick to add laundry charges to each occupied room—no one would be able to detect them. If food service was falling below its revenue target, "room service" orders could be sent to a selection of patients without an order, and be added to the bill. Short of a special investigation, it would be impossible to detect these changes, especially given the labyrinthian nature of the hospital billing and receivables processes. An analogy for hospital bureaucracy has been proposed: a hotel in Greece serves only tour groups from Japan. It accepts payment only in Russian currency. All billing statements are prepared in German, and are routed through a French billing service. All payments must be made to a French bank, but only in rubles. These arrangements would roughly equate to hospital billing practices in the United States, certainly prior to the arrival of prospective payment. What DRGs do is pay a set amount for each patient based on the admitting diagnosis, period. For the manager performance is not based on higher revenues. The new challenge becomes figuring out how to provide the necessary care for less money than the DRG payment provides the hospital. The alteration in incentives imposed on hospitals by the prospective DRG-based payment system has had some measurable impact in slowing the rate of inflation of inpatient hospital expenditures, for both government and private payers. Writing about DRGs in 1985, Walter McClure of the Center for Policy Studies in Minneapolis said:

> Medicare, the biggest purchaser, . . . has moved from a totally disastrous buy wrong strategy to an only semidisastrous buy wrong strategy. Because the new strategy pays on price rather than cost, it is demonstrably superior to the old strategy. But it gives patients neither means nor incentives to choose high quality efficient providers. It is therefore forced, predictably, to arbitrarily freeze prices and utilization rates, and it will do much mischief to patients (especially sick patients), to efficient quality providers and to the ability of other purchasers to buy right. It will be necessary to move Medicare beyond DRGs.[34]

In shifting to prospective payment and DRGs, Congress can nonetheless credit itself with having undertaken a step in healthcare reform that could qualify as intelligent.

However, just five years after enacting the new prospective payment system for Medicare, the Congress passed Public Law 100-351, a catastrophic health-insurance bill for the elderly. It was signed into law by President Bush in July 1988. Despite the lessons to be learned from nearly a quarter-century of legislative adventures akin to Alice's experiences in Wonderland, Congress had not yet absorbed the most fundamental lesson of all about health reform: Do not pump more resources into medical care unless or until there has been a radical restructuring and reconstruction of the American healthcare system. What Bert Seidman told Congress in 1979 about catastrophic health-insurance legislation held true of P.L.100-351: "What is conspicuously absent . . . is an understanding of the basic economics of the health care industry." Consider this lesson as expressed in the words of Walter McClure in 1975:

> The quantity, quality and style of medical care are indefinitely expansible. The medical care system can legitimately absorb every dollar society will make available to it . . . inventive American science and technology can endlessly elaborate the possibilities. The final check on what gets done is the dollars available.[35]

The trick in 1988 was to pour additional billions into the coffers of the American medical guild and its workshops without increasing the federal deficit. This was to be accomplished by the imposition of a "surtax" to offset whatever costs the catastrophic insurance would generate. The federal treasury was to be protected by the device of distributing the total annual cost of the catastrophic protection to all Medicare beneficiaries, equally, through the addition of a "surtax" in the required amount to the billings sent out each quarter for Part B Medicare coverage. It might be a dollar, or three dollars, or a hundred dollars per quarter, or even per month. Congress made no firm predictions about future costs, satisfied that the federal government would suffer no additional expense. When America's senior citizens recognized what the Congress had done, placing the heaviest burden on older Americans who would probably account for most of the expenditures generated by this law, the reaction was strong enough to cause the Congress to repeal P.L. 100–351. The vehicle of repeal was P.L. 101–234, the Medicare Catastrophic Repeal Act, passed on December 13, 1989. The initial law was never implemented.

For at least the twenty-five-year period 1963 to 1988, Congress undertook healthcare reform efforts that were rooted in two major erroneous assumptions: (a) throwing more dollars into medical care will alone cure the illness that threatens the national economy; and (b) regardless of the fact that all of the horses have left, there is some purpose to be served in spending large sums to secure the barn doors behind them.

The stories about how the federal government has erred in purchasing even such mundane items such as hammers, toilet seats, and ashtrays pale to insignificance when compared with the federal performance in making arrangements to provide medical-care coverage to the variety of people who are currently entitled to such benefits.

The Value in Buying Right

There are some outstanding examples of the benefits to be gained from "buying right" when it comes to healthcare—benefits to both purchasers and patients. Twenty years ago, the Health Benefits division of the California Public Employees Retirement System (CALPERS) offered its clients throughout California a choice among several indemnity insurance plans (Blue Cross, Blue Shield, Aetna, Prudential, etc.) and the Kaiser prepaid group practice plan, now known as an HMO. Kaiser had perhaps 20 percent of the eligible beneficiaries, and the indemnities had the rest. Ten years later, all of the private-sector indemnity plans were gone, and the CALPERS clients had a choice among a half-dozen or more HMOs—depending upon the geographic region—and one indemnity-type plan sponsored by CALPERS itself. The latter option, selected by a small number of CALPERS clients, has required the largest payroll deduction for the beneficiary, and it has nonetheless represented a consistent financial drain for CALPERS. In a report dated June 11, 1996, the Congressional Budget Office included a six-year history of annual increases or decreases in CALPERS premiums:

1990	+17%
1991	+11%
1992	+ 6%
1993	+ 1%
1994	− 1%
1995	− 4%

Through intelligent purchasing practices, CALPERS drove out the high-ticket indemnity plans that did no more than handle payments to service providers, and replaced them with a collection of direct-service, well managed, efficient HMOs. The HMOs are competing among themselves to attract and hold CALPERS clients—competing to provide the best quality of medical care and the highest level of service to the CALPERS beneficiaries. Buying right can and does pay handsome dividends, in this instance saving the pension fund millions of dollars, and keeping the clients highly satisfied with their health coverage options. CALPERS has significant purchasing leverage in the California market, and it has used it wisely and well.

Annual federal expenditures for medical care currently constitute about 40 percent of the total annual national outlay, now running at over $1 trillion a year. The federal expenditures include the Federal Employees Health Benefits Program (FEHBP), CHAMPUS, Veterans Administration health programs, Medicare, Medicaid, CDC, NIH, military hospitals and treatment facilities worldwide, and Public Health Service programs including grant assistance to neighborhood and rural health centers and other health facilities. If the federal government used this enormous purchasing leverage wisely and well—if it spent this $400 billion dollars annually using a "buy right" strategy—the savings would be astounding, and the pressure for reform would be profound, forcing changes in the present healthcare system that must occur if the nation is to avoid eventual economic disaster. However, the federal government appears to be bending its every effort to buy health benefits the wrong way at every available opportunity. Although poor federal purchasing patterns are endemic throughout the programs listed above, the largest purchasing leverage in the constellation of federal health programs belongs to Medicare, therefore a description of the follies evident in Medicare purchasing will serve as a general illustration of the problems manifest in each specific program.

The Costs of Buying Wrong

For calendar 1996, Medicare expenditures totaled about $200 billion, for a beneficiary population of about 38 million people. The annual per capita expenditure for 1996 would therefore be about $5,200. A rough monthly average per capita cost for the entire country can be derived by dividing $5,200 by twelve, which results in a United States Per Capita Cost (USPCC) of $433 for calendar 1996. The Health Care Financing Administration (HCFA) is the federal agency responsible for Medicare, and it has a far more complex formula for calculating the USPCC. Anyone with the courage to try to understand HCFA's formula would quickly decide that it is virtually incomprehensible. It reminds me of a philosophy professor who enjoyed telling his students that the great German geniuses in his field prided themselves in being adept at writing philosophy so that no one could understand it. HCFA may have passed this mark with the USPCC formula.

The USPCC combined number for Parts A and B of Medicare for the aged category for 1995 was $400.52, of which $251.61 was Part A and $148.91 was Part B. In November 1995, HCFA revised its 1996 calculation of the USPCCs to reflect a cost inflation of 10.1 percent, therefore the combined USPCC for aged, non-ESRD was $440.57. Note that the difference between the foregoing rough calculation of $433 and the subsequent official USPCC approximation of $440.57 is $7.57—or about 1.7 percent. This would appear to be close enough for government work; however, one of the pivotal lessons to be learned about Medicare is the significance of scale. With 38 million beneficiaries as the multiplier, a difference of $7.57 in USPCC, i.e., in per beneficiary per month costs, would add up to $3.5 billion during one twelve-month period. Seemingly small sums of money end up making huge differences within a program the size of Medicare, expending over $200 billion annually in federal tax dollars. Why is the USPCC for Medicare continuing to escalate at an annual rate of 10 percent or more during the same period in which CALPERS premiums have been *declining*? The geniuses in charge of HCFA during the tenure of President Clinton happen to believe that HMOs cannot solve the cost inflation that has been ravaging Medicare since the 1980s. Under this leadership, therefore, HCFA has managed to maintain very high rates of increase in per capita expenditures during a period in which most large private employers (and public programs such as CALPERS) have experienced stable or declining health-benefits costs. In a June 1996 report on Medicare spending, the Congressional Budget Office (CBO) said this:

> [T]he striking difference in the recent experience of the private and public sectors clearly suggests that private health plans have achieved more effective control over spending than has Medicare. . . . In exchange for slower spending growth, employers and employees in the private sector have accepted more management of their health services and restrictions on their choice of providers. Most Medicare beneficiaries, by contrast, are still enrolled in the traditional fee-for-service Medicare program, which represents a type of unmanaged health plan that is fast disappearing in the employment-based health insurance market.[36]

In 1996 HCFA was "reorganized" in a manner that buried the previously independent HMO contracting office deep inside the division that runs the huge Medicare fee-for-service operations. Prepaid "risk" contracts are anathema to fee-for-service adherents within HCFA, for the reason that their jobs would be threatened by a surge of enrollment into HMO plans, if for no other reason. Had the example of CALPERS and the large private employers been emulated during the past four years, the taxpayers might have saved over $50 billion. The failure to effectively push an HMO strategy for Medicare has resulted in an unconscionable and indefensible waste of society's treasure at the hands of HCFA officials.

Viewed otherwise, the May 1998 CBO report entitled *Long-Term Budgetary Pressures and Policy Options* uses an average annual growth rate of 8.5 percent for Medicare payments between 1997 and 2008, and cautions about "rising per-enrollee costs of health care," noting that "no policy in force promises to check the open-ended entitlements for health care." At this rate, total annual Medicare expenditures would increase from the 1997 level of $304 billion to $745.8 billion in 2008—more than a doubling within the next ten years. During the next ten years (i.e., 1999 through 2008), total expenditures for the period on Medicare beneficiaries alone would add up to $5.3 trillion, about five times current annual expenditures for the entire American population. If the rate of increase could be held to 2 percent, as has been achieved by CALPERS and thousands of other major employers, total Medicare expenditures for the same ten-year period would be $3.46 trillion, nearly two trillion dollars ($1.84 trillion) less than the CBO now projects spending. This startling difference should provide a clear sense of the huge stakes involved in the reconstruction of the present medical care system. The society has both a HCFA administration with an erroneous view of the potential value of HMOs as a tool of reform, and a Congress without much of a clue to thank for this abject and ongoing waste of nearly 2 trillion dollars in public monies over the next ten years.

Starting around 1985, and continuing to the present, the HCFA has contracted with HMOs on a restricted basis to enroll Medicare beneficiaries. These "risk" contracts were authorized and directed by the Congress under P.L. 97-248, the Tax Equity and Fiscal Responsibility Act (TEFRA). The basis of payment under these contracts has been a rate entitled the Adjusted Average Per Capita Cost (AAPCC), with separate rates being calculated each year for each county in the United States, for Parts A and B, and for both aged and disabled categories. Every year, HCFA publishes a new ratebook containing the county-specific rates that result from the complex calculations.

The key defect in HCFA's formulas for arriving at AAPCC rates is evident in the following excerpt from a description of HCFA's methodology:

> [A]n adjustment based solely on a historical cost relationship would not be sufficient to estimate the contract year cost relationship between the county and the nation. *Since the AAPCC should be the best estimate of fee-for-service reimbursements in the county in the contract year,* another adjustment is made for the changes in the hospital payment provisions. PPS provisions are applied only under Part A, so the Part B USPCC is not affected by this additional adjustment. (Emphasis added)

If the rate paid under a risk contract represents the "best estimate of fee-for-service reimbursement in the county in the contract year," the rate is essentially a reflection of how the fee-based physician free barons have been behaving within that community. If there are two thousand physicians in a community taking care of the entire population; if a Kaiser plan moves in, builds a hospital, and enrolls half of the employed people in town, but no Medicare beneficiaries; and if the two thousand physicians decide they like the community, and, despite the loss of half of the employed citizens as patients, none leave; then the non-Kaiser members in the community are going to receive an average of twice as much medical care as they did before Kaiser came to town. The unnecessary medical and surgical care will fall heaviest on the Medicare folks, because Medicare reimbursement represents the most attractive revenue source, in that the federal government has the deepest pockets.

It is worthy of special note that, in the HCFA description of its AAPCC methodology, the word "cost" is used throughout as equivalent to the words "reimbursement" or "expenditure." In fact, HCFA's seemingly ingenious but seriously defective AAPCC formula contains no calculation of "cost," but simply assumes that the word means "the sum total of what has been spent." USPCC should properly be USPCE, with the "E" standing for "expenditure."

This most glaring defect in HCFA's "actuarial" rate-making scheme is clearly in evidence in the published "rate tables." It is a defect that may in part explain why the Medicare program has been so retarded in following the example of major private employers, who have been using HMOs to gain effective control over runaway medical care costs. The impact that this glaring defect is having can be seen vividly by comparing the 1996 aged AAPCC rate for one county—Loving, Texas—with the USPCC rates for the same year:

Loving, Texas—Calendar 1996

Part A—Aged		$698.08
Part B—Aged		183.27
	Total:	$881.27

USPCC—Calendar 1996

Part A—Aged		$277.02
Part A—Aged		163.95
	Total:	$440.97

The difference between these two rates is $440.30 per capita per month, or $5,284 per capita per year. Applying the lesson of scale, if all Medicare beneficiaries were enrolled in HMOs under the 1996 Aged AAPCC rate for Loving, Texas, total annual expenditures for Medicare would be doubled—rising from the current $200 billion to more than $400 billion for that one year.

How is it possible that Congress and the HCFA administrator could, for the one program that holds out any hope of controlling Medicare expenditures, support a rate-making procedure, year in and year out, that is so fundamentally flawed that it pays twice as much for an enrolled Medicare beneficiary who lives in Loving, Texas, as is currently being spent per capita on 38 million Medicare beneficiaries in the nation as a whole?

How is it possible that HCFA could publish AAPCC rates for Loving, Texas, and for Richmond County, New York, that are double the per capita outlay under the inefficient fee-for-service Medicare program, and yet not recognize that there is something terribly wrong?

Many thoughtful people in the HMO business have understood for as long as a decade that something is very wrong with HCFA's rate-making scheme, and have pondered the question whether the glaring defect in the HCFA methodology is the result of viciousness or of stupidity on the part of the Congress, the HCFA administrator, and the actuaries. There can be no middle ground—the source of this defect has to be one or the other. Purposeful sabotage of the rate-making procedures for TEFRA "risk" contracts would certainly retard the growth of enrollment into HMOs. Such slowed HMO growth in Medicare has been of enormous financial benefit to the physician free barons in fee-based practice, who are among the top contributors to congressional officeholders. Holding back the shift of beneficiaries into HMOs also protects the existing HCFA bureaucracy by not disturbing its ongoing functions in contracting with fiscal intermediaries for the piecework payment of $200 billion in claims annually to 680,000 fee-for-service physicians throughout the nation, and to 6,500 hospitals, most of them under the DRG program. The huge and sprawling HCFA administrative apparatus would rapidly disappear if all Medicare beneficiaries elected membership in an HMO as the way to obtain their benefits.

It should be clear that the defect distorting the AAPCC rates promulgated by HCFA arises principally from the folly of using actual fee-for-service expenditure experience within each specific county as a basis for deriving a prospective rate for the TEFRA "risk" contracts. There are counties in America in which, by age sixty-five, 70 percent of females have had their uterus removed; and there are counties in which less than 10 percent of women have had a hysterectomy by the age of sixty-five. This wild and radical variation in the incidence of a single surgical procedure, which physician free barons grandly attribute to differences in "practice style," is explained chiefly by the presence or absence of gynecology surgeons, and by the relative availability of surgical beds. It is also evident from the brute facts about radical variations in the practices of American physicians that the greater the concentration of physicians and surgeons in a community, the greater the expenditure for medical care will be in that community. If the nationwide ratio of physicians to population is currently 240 per 100,000, as the Pew Commission has established; and if in a specific county it is 480 per 100,000, it is reasonable to conclude that per capita expenditures for medical care in that county will be twice as high as overall Medicare per capita expenditures.

By using county-specific fee-for-service *expenditures* in the AAPCC ratemaking formula, the HCFA actuaries have created a fundamentally irrational, obviously wrongheaded, and generally unworkable payment scheme for these contracts. To illustrate this point, a plan with a TEFRA "risk" contract enrolling Aged Medicare beneficiaries in Culebra, Puerto Rico, in 1996 would have been paid $39.32 for Part A and $88.12 for Part B, or a total of $127.44 per enrollee per month. This is *$753.83 less* per person per month than would be paid in Loving, Texas. In other words, based on the 1996 AAPCC ratebook, HCFA paid 7 *times as much* for an Aged Medicare beneficiary who lived in Loving, Texas as they would have paid for the same Aged Medicare beneficiary had they been living in Culebra, Puerto Rico. How is it possible that HCFA could calculate and publish rates of payment which *vary by 700 percent,* based solely on the county of residence of the Medicare beneficiary? When pressed forcefully in 1985 about this fundamental irrationality and its destructive consequences for the "risk" contracts and for the Medicare program, Guy King, then the HCFA actuary, could only blame the Congress. He was merely following the terms that Congress had set forth in P.L.97-248 (TEFRA), and his hands were tied. It has been over a decade since that conversation occurred, and Guy King has now moved on to a position in private industry. Nothing has changed at HCFA, however, to correct the glaring defect in its AAPCC ratemaking scheme.

The most frustrating dimension of this specific congressional and executive branch folly is that a very simple and straightforward methodology already exists within HCFA that could be applied to deriving the appropriate rates to pay under TEFRA "risk" contracts. The Medicare physician fee schedule used by HCFA to reimburse fee-for-service physicians is subjected to a "geographic adjustment factor," which HCFA derives from analyses of changes in the Medical Economic Index (MEI) and other general price indices. The intent in applying these adjustments is to reflect differences in the cost of doing business, and in the cost of living, between or among different geographic areas across the nation. HCFA publishes its physician fee schedules reflecting the geographic adjustment for each specific "locality." The variations from one "locality" to another within a given state are fairly slight. In Florida, for example, HCFA has cut the state up into four distinct "localities." The variation in the HCFA fee schedule for ICD Code 19380— "revise breast reconstruction"—between locality #1 and locality #2 was 3 percent, with locality #1 having the lower rate—$561.60 versus $580.35.

As an example of the simplified approach that could be used in lieu of an AAPCC, assume that expenditures in locality #1 were "average," and that the rate to be paid for 1996 to a "risk" contractor in that locality would therefore be $440.97—i.e., the USPCC for Parts A and B, Aged. The rate for "risk" contracts covering locality #2 would then be 3 percent higher, or $454.20. This level of variation in rates would be reasonable, manageable, and entirely consistent with a good faith effort by HCFA to detect differences in *basic costs* between and among different geographic areas. On the face of this example, there would seem to be no legitimate reason for HCFA to have created the present tortured and perverse AAPCC ratemaking methodology, which HCFA actuaries are now using to derive rates with ludicrous variations, unexplained by anything other than how radically out of control the fee-based free barons may be in one community as compared with another. HCFA's only handy excuse for this ongoing atrocious and clearly unactuarial behavior is that Congress is making them do it.

If "risk" payments were based directly on the USPCC, and varied within a narrow range around that national calculation, HMOs in all parts of the country could, and most probably would, compete for these Medicare contracts, and the Medicare program could thereby benefit from the increased control of expenditures that CALPERS and thousands of large private-sector employers have been realizing over the past five years or more. Of course, the free barons of the medical guild and their AMA lobbyists would be most unhappy and upset, because the biggest, best, and truly bottomless pot of gold remaining available to them—HCFA fee-for-service reimbursements—would turn up with a firm new bottom, and would soon prove to be unavailable. This is what occurred at CALPERS ten years ago. And this explains why, at present, the medical guild is investing heavily in efforts everywhere to prevent any further HMO penetration of the fee-for-service "market share," with the lucrative Medicare program being their primary concern.

Analysis of the HCFA-produced AAPCC ratebooks for the years 1985 through 1996 yields many marvels other than the aforementioned glaring defect in methodology. For example, consider the following "brute facts" drawn from the 1996 AAPCC rate tables and Pew Commission reports:

1. As reported by the PEW Commission, of the fifty states and the District of Columbia, only *twenty states* have 40 percent or more of all their "patient care physicians" (as defined by the Pew Commission) engaged in primary care, with the highest percentage—56.3 percent—belonging to Iowa.

2. There are *twenty-eight counties* in the 1996 HCFA ratebook with AAPCC rates for Part A, aged that are in excess of $400, constituting the highest rates in the land.

3. Not a single one of these *twenty-eight counties* with the highest Part A AAPCC rates is located in one of the *twenty states* having over 40 percent of their physicians in primary care.

4. The state with the lowest percentage of its physicians in primary care—27.6 percent, less than half the percentage in Iowa—is *Louisiana.*

5. One-fourth, 25 percent, of the *twenty-eight counties* with 1996 Part A AAPCC rates exceeding $400 are located in *Louisiana,* with its scarcity of primary physicians.

It all fits very neatly. This analysis establishes the point that the Part A aged AAPCC rate varies inversely with the percentage of primary-care physicians working within a county. The lower the former, the higher the latter, and vice versa.

A "brute fact" confirming this point is that the ten states having the *lowest* Part A aged AAPCC rates for 1996 had the *highest number of doctors engaged in primary care,* as a percentage of all "patient-care physicians." In these ten states, an average of 49.5 percent of all "patient-care physicians" were engaged in primary care, with Iowa having the highest percentage, as noted above. It is fascinating to note that eight of these ten states with the lowest AAPCC rates had an Osteopathic medical school located within their borders; and in all eight states, not less than 40 percent of all primary-care physicians were Doctors of Osteopathy (D.O.s), not Doctors of Medicine (M.D.s). This latter analysis points to the conclusion that the Part A aged AAPCC rate varies inversely with the proportion of primary care physicians who are D.O.s—the lower the former, the higher the latter, and vice versa. The most reasonable explanation for this conclusion is that the D.O.s who have been practicing in these states long enough to have affected these data were trained in an entirely different manner than were most primary doctors holding M.D. degrees, and their practice patterns are therefore entirely different. In this instance, the evidence is clear that the D.O.s exhibit practice patterns that rely far less on hospital-based or hospital-intensive care than do their M.D. colleagues.

Another remarkable finding from an analysis of HCFA's 1985 to 1996 AAPCC ratebooks is that enormous variations have occurred during these years in the rates for certain counties that cannot be accounted for by changes in the morbidity indices, but can be explained by the brute fact that the physician suppliers have purposefully raised the levels of demand. Here are some examples:

County	1985 Part A Aged AAPCC	1996 Part A Aged AAPCC	Difference
Thockmorton, Tx.	$184	$163	− 12%
Loving, Tx.	$118	$881	+745%
Richmond, N.Y.	$172	$758	+441%
Bronx, N.Y.	$184	$734	+399%
New York, N.Y.	$180	$715	+397%

It is notable that, on the list of 50 counties with the highest Part A aged AAPCC rates for 1996, only 11 had made that same list in 1985. That is, there are 39 "newcomer" counties on the 1996 top-50 list. The number-one county on the 1985 list did not make the 1996 list. Dade County, Florida, which was number 7 on the 1985 list; Washington, D.C., which was number 15; and Los Angeles, which was number 16 are no longer in the top-50 in

1996. Since these were among the most attractive places to develop a Medicare "risk" contract a dozen years ago, because they had high AAPCC rates, the subsequent penetration by well-run HMOs has been very high in certain of these counties, and this has driven the gross per capita Medicare expenditures down dramatically enough that the AAPCC rates—heavily based as they are on Medicare fee-for-service expenditures in a specific county—have fallen significantly year after year relative to Medicare outlays in most other counties, where fee-for-service reimbursement predominates.

At first glance, the phenomenon of falling AAPCC rates where "risk" contract enrollment has been high may seem to represent a success for HCFA. However, what is in fact occurring amounts to a *reductio ad absurdam*: the initial rate paid to "risk" contractors was exorbitantly high in certain counties; contracting plans proceeded to enroll 50 percent or more of the Medicare beneficiaries in those counties; because the HCFA rate-making methodology is using fee-for-service expenditure within a county to derive the AAPCC rate, as the fee-for-service outlays begin to decrease in these counties, because beneficiaries are enrolled in HMOs, the pendulum swing produced by the HMO penetration in those counties is influenced by this same defect, only in the opposite direction. The HCFA methodology then produces an AAPCC rate that is *well below the USPCC*. As an example, if the 1996 USPCC for both Parts A and B, Medicare aged was $440, then Dade County's 1996 AAPCC rate of $335 for these members was 31 percent lower than the USPCC. How is it possible to explain this outcome other than by finding that the HCFA methodology is designed to insure the failure of the TEFRA "risk" contract initiative? After all, many in HCFA leadership positions strongly believe that the fee-for-service reimbursement program is "their" program, and that those who support "risk" contracts are interlopers. In any event, there is no other legitimate conclusion to be drawn from an analysis of HCFA's rate-making methodology for Medicare "risk" contracts than that the scheme is fundamentally and irreparably flawed. AAPCC needs to be scrapped and replaced by a simpler, more straightforward method using a broad national baseline such as the USPCC as the principal yardstick for determining "risk" contract rates.

The glaring defect in the calculation of Medicare rates for HMOs is rooted in an erroneous assumption on the part of the Congress, or on the part of HCFA officials, or both. Especially in light of the fact of a stubborn refusal by all federal players—Congress and the administration—to address this defect, the possibility has been alluded to that the erroneous assumption may also be a pernicious assumption. Whatever the truth is, this persistent flaw represents a tragic and unconscionable waste of national treasure, and a social sin of the worst kind.

Notes

1. Anne R. Somers, *Health Care in Transition: Directions for the Future* (Chicago: Hospital Research and Education Trust, 1969), p. 36.

2. R. Stevens, *American Medicine and the Public Interest* (New Haven, Conn.: Yale University Press, 1971), p. 510.

3. J. Wennberg, *Report on Health Care in Vermont*, Northern New England Regional Medical Program (December 1971), p. 34.

4. L. P. Williams, *How to Avoid Unnecessary Surgery* (Los Angeles: Nash, 1971), p. 21.

5. P. Starr, *The Social Transformation of American Medicine: The Rise of a Sovereign Profession and the Making of a Vast Industry* (New York: BasicBooks, 1982).

6. Ibid., pp. 268–69.

7. Ibid., pp. 375–85.

8. J. Wennberg, "Which Rate Is Right?" *New England Journal of Medicine* 314 (January 30, 1986): 311.

9. Ibid., p. 311.

10. J. Krakower, "Review of U.S. Medical School Finances, 1994–95," *Journal of the American Medical Association* 276, no. 9 (September 4, 1996): 724.

11. E. Ginzberg, "The Restructuring of U.S. Health Care," *Inquiry* (Fall 1985), p. 274.

12. B. Seidman, Congressional Testimony, Senate Finance Committee, March 28, 1979, p. 11.

13. Pew Health Professions Commission, *Critical Challenges: Revitalizing the Health Professions for the Twenty-first Century*, 2d Report, December 1995, p. xvi.

14. S. Block, Nancy Clark-Chiarelli, Antoinette S. Peters, and Judith D. Singer, "Academia's Chilly Climate for Primary Care," *Journal of the American Medical Association* 276, no. 9 (September 4, 1996): 677–82.

15. SOSSUS, *Surgery in the United States: A Summary Report of the Study on Surgical Services for the United States*, conducted under the joint auspices of the American College of Surgeons and the American Surgical Association, 1975.

16. J. Morrow and A. B. Edwards, "U. S. Health Manpower Policy: Will the Benefits Justify the Costs?" *Journal of Medical Education* 51 (1976): 791.

17. D. C. Williams, "Surgeons and Surgery in Rhode Island, 1970 and 1977," *New England Journal of Medicine* 305, no. 22 (November 26, 1981): 1319–23.

18. A. N. Whitehead, *Science and the Modern World* (New York: Free Press, 1957), p. 55.

19. Ibid., p. 50.

20. I. McWhinney, "Family Medicine as a Science," *Journal of Family Practice* 7, no. 1 (1978): 54.

21. Ibid.

22. K. Ernst, "Integrating Quality Diabetes Care into the Evolution of Health Care," *On the Cutting Edge* (Winter 1996): 16.

23. McWhinney, "Family Medicine as a Science," pp. 55–56.

24. Ibid., pp. 56–57.

25. I. McWhinney, "Family Medicine in Perspective," *New England Journal of Medicine* 293, no. 4 (July 24, 1975): 177.

26. Starr, *The Social Transformation of American Medicine*, p. 370.

27. Ibid., p. 399.

28. Editor, *Fortune*, January 1970.

29. Starr, *The Social Transformation of American Medicine*, p. 397.

30. Editor, *National Journal* 8 (October 16, 1976): 1460.

31. Starr, *The Social Transformation of American Medicine*, p. 376.

32. Ibid., p. 402.

33. Spencer Rich, *Washington Post*, February 27, 1987.

34. W. McClure, "Buying Right: The Consequences of Glut," *Business and Health* (September 1985): 44.

35. W. McClure, "The Medical Care System Under National Health Insurance: Four Models that Might Work and Their Prospects," *Interstudy* (September 1975): 12–13.

36. Congressional Budget Office, *Trends in Health Spending by the Private Sector and Medicare*, report to Congress, June 11, 1996.

5.

What Should Be Done? Reconstruction as a Necessity

The claim that American medicine represents "the best medicine in the world" has been repeated so often that many people in this country accept it as accurate. The brute facts are quite otherwise. The medical care system in this country is badly broken—so broken in fact that it now represents a major threat to the continued economic health and survival of the society. As for the impact of this fiscally disabled system on the physical health of Americans, life expectancy statistics provide a significant indicator of the effectiveness of the medical care system upon which a population depends. How does the United States compare with other countries of the world when it comes to life expectancy? *The World Health Statistics Annual* for 1990 has reported that the 20 countries with the highest life expectancy at birth are ranked as follows:[1]

1.	Japan	76.2
2.	Greece	74.3
3.	Sweden	74.2
4.	Switzerland	74.1
5.	Netherlands	73.7
6.	Israel	73.6

7.	Spain	73.4
8.	Canada	73.4
9.	Italy	73.3
10.	Australia	73.2
11.	Iceland	73.2
12.	France	72.9
13.	Britain	72.7
14.	Germany	72.6
15.	Denmark	72.2
16.	Costa Rica	72.1
17.	Austria	72.1
18.	Norway	72.1
19.	Cuba	72.0
20.	United States	71.6

How is it possible that a nation with "the best medical care in the world," and most certainly the most expensive medical care in the world, could be at the bottom of the top-twenty list in terms of life expectancy?

Comparing the statistics for the United States with those for the top nation in life expectancy—Japan—provides some even more unsettling insight: As aging proceeds, Japanese citizens gain statistical ground on U.S. citizens in terms of life expectancy. For example, at birth a Japanese infant has a 6.4 percent life expectancy (LE) advantage over an American infant, with an expectation of 4.6 years of additional life. As aging proceeds, this Japanese advantage consistently increases:[2]

Age	LE/Japan	LE/United States	Years	Percent
15	61.8	57.7	+4.1	+7.1%
45	33.2	30.5	+2.7	+8.9%
65	16.5	15	+1.5	+10%

How is it possible that, as aging goes on, American citizens, living in a nation that has been led to believe that it has "the best medical care in the world," are progressively losing life expectancy as they get older, compared with the citizens of Japan? How is it possible that, with each passing year, Americans are dying sooner than the Japanese, despite the fact that we are spending a far greater percentage of our gross domestic product on medical care?

This is possible because American medicine has organized itself on the basis of a scheme of ideas that is fundamentally in error, and is therefore propelling the practice of medicine along pathways that lead directly to outcomes shown in the foregoing statistical comparisons of life expectancy. Bluntly stated, America does not have "the best medical care in the world," although its annual per capita expenditures on medical care are second to none. The authority, prestige, and power that American physicians and their medical guild have garnered within this society make it extremely unlikely that what ought to be done to fix what is wrong with this major dimension of American life will in fact be done. While it may be difficult or even impossible to make any significant change in the current medical scheme of ideas, or in the organizational structures it spawned, it may nonetheless be useful to set forth the reforms that ought to be enacted to reconstruct the present scheme in ways that will repair what is broken, and thereby enable Americans to achieve health status outcomes that would justify our claim to superiority. In considering what ought to be done, it would be wise for federal legislators, in particular, to bear in mind one of the insightful sayings of Yogi Berra: "If you don't know where you're going, you may end up somewhere else."

Reconstruction in American medical and health care must occur in six specific aspects:

1. The reorganization of medical education and practice
2. The reorganization of medical information
3. The reorganization of membership plans
4. The organization of evaluative clinical science
5. The reorganization of economic incentives
6. The reorganization of competition

These six aspects of a thoroughgoing reconstruction are interdependent, which is to say that if any one of them is left out of the reform scheme, the whole change that is required cannot be accomplished. The relationships between and among the six enumerated aspects of American medicine are at least as significant as the distinctions between any one of the aspects and another of those aspects. As with the building of a skyscraper, none of these essential structural elements can be overlooked or omitted without undermining the entire effort at reconstruction and reorganization. Let's review these ingredients of fruitful change in the American medical cosmos, and in its currently dominant scheme of ideas:

Reorganization of Medical Education and Medical Practice

Medical education and medical practice need to be turned on their heads. The beginning of fruitful reconstruction requires the recognition of a fundamental fact: There is no possibility of reforming the American healthcare system in effective ways unless the ratio of licensed, practicing physicians to the consuming population can be brought into reasonable balance; and unless the proportions between physicians providing primary care and all other physicians—so-called specialists—can be radically altered within a short period of time. The fundamental problem that must be squarely faced by anyone seeking to make significant and enduring changes in the clinical efficacy or in the economics of the contemporary medical marketplace is with the kind, the number, and the distribution of medical doctors in this society. This stubborn reality is rarely mentioned in the volumes of expert analysis pouring out of our universities and "think tanks," yet it defines a principal part of the context within which meaningful and lasting reform must be discovered. Neglect of this brute fact will undermine every theory of "health reform" that overlooks its importance in any realistic consideration of what ought to be done to ameliorate current patterns of providing medical and healthcare services in this country.

This means that the output of the 125 fully accredited medical schools in this country must be changed in at least three significant ways:

(a) the number of medical graduates must be reduced dramatically during the next decade or longer;

(b) the kind of physicians being produced by these schools must change radically; and,

(c) a revolution must occur in the preparation of physicians to practice family medicine.

What is called for is nothing short of a new "Flexner Report," specifying the ways and means to reconstruct basic and graduate medical education and to redefine the criteria for selecting medical students.

Reversing the Medical Center

At the dawn of the twenty-first century, American medicine requires the equivalent of a Copernican revolution, i.e., a complete reversal of centers in the medical cosmos. A consensus evolved around the turn of the twentieth century that specialized knowledge would be superior in importance to general medical knowledge—the more specialized the knowledge, the more important. And the most important of all medical knowledge would be that related to high-tech surgical practice at the very top of the medical world. Assumptions about the order of things in the cosmos influence theory, define our logic and form the patterns for thought and action. It is important to recognize that the most commonplace assumptions held within American medicine today continue to be wrong.

The erroneous and largely unexposed scheme of ideas that has guided American medicine during the twentieth century accounts for the following litany of aberrations evident today:

- the status of primary-care physicians as second- or third-class players in the medical hierarchy;

- the virtual absence of evaluative clinical science;

- the primitive nature of the medical information system;

- the radical variations in medical practice, attributed by the profession to differences in "style";

- the consistent breaching of the Hippocratic oath through the widespread performance of inappropriate or unnecessary procedures and treatment;

- the medical guild's persistent support of fee-for-service as being the essential factor in freedom of choice for the patient.

These aberrations, which ought to be a source of immense embarrassment to every physician, are all reflective of the unacknowledged, unexamined and erroneous scheme of ideas—the engine of contemporary American medicine. In science, general knowledge is of the highest order of importance, being essential to achieve the integration of all special knowledge. American medicine has it exactly backwards. The *Flexner Report* led directly to the subversion of the medical generalist, and consequently to the perversion of medical epistemology and of the medical community of inquiry. Flexner's heritage is 125 fully accredited medical schools, all existing in a Wonderland.

Since the early 1970s, Ian McWhinney, M.D., has been teaching and writing about the calamities for organized medicine resulting from its systematic denigration of the generalist physician. During the past two decades, his efforts to alert his profession about its blunder can accurately be described as those of a voice crying out in the wilderness. In a 1975 article, he made the following observations:

> The Flexner reforms accelerated two processes: the concentration of both medical care and medical education in the hospital. . . . The hospital by its very nature tends to separate the disease from the man and the man from his environment. It is not surprising, therefore, that the medicine of this century has been the medicine of entities rather than the medicine of relations and that modern medicine has, as John Ryle remarked in 1948, neglected etiology in its widest sense. How many physicians going into practice have found themselves totally unprepared by their training for their encounter with illness outside the hospital! . . . Many general practitioners found that their world view was being gradually changed by their experience. They saw many illnesses that could not be fitted into the neat categories that they had learned. They learned that illness is intimately related to the personality and life experience of the patient. They learned the inseparability of patient and environment. This change in world view can be likened to a change in visual gestalt. The general practitioner, trained to see illness in terms of the figure, began gradually to see both figure and ground. *He found that to understand illness it is necessary also to understand its context.*[3] (Emphasis added)

Ian McWhinney was telling us, twenty years ago, that, given the way that medical epistemology is now structured, the education being offered by schools of medicine can never be fully coherent; and, given the way that the medical cosmos is now structured, the outcomes for patients can never be fully coherent. He did not add the equally true and significant fact that the way the economic reward system is largely structured in medicine, the outcomes for either the physician or the patient can never be fully coherent.

The Importance of Generalism in Medicine

The solution to these problems of incoherence requires a reversal of the centers in the medical world, based on a recognition and acceptance of the irreducible fact that the general point of view is the most important in medical science and practice. In her book *Primary Care: Concept, Evaluation and Policy,* Barbara Starfield provides an excellent definition of "primary care":

> The delivery of first-contact medicine; the assumption of longitudinal responsibility for the patient, regardless of the presence or absence of disease; and the integration of physical, psychological, and social aspects of health.[4]

All "special" aspects of medical science and practice must be brought under the central vision of the medical generalist engaged in primary care. Given a reconstruction like this, evaluative clinical science will thereby be afforded a realistic opportunity to prevail.

Mismanaging Diabetes

A digression is in order here, to present a concrete example of the untoward and unacceptable outcomes that society is currently experiencing as the direct result of the topsy-turvy epistemology and scheme of ideas driving medical practice in America today.

Diabetes Mellitus (DM) is a prevalent disease in the United States. It inhibits the body's ability to produce or to utilize insulin, a hormone normally produced by the pancreas. The resulting high blood-sugar levels damage blood vessels, which, over time, can lead to impaired circulation.

Since high blood sugar damages blood vessels generally, diabetes contributes to many medical problems, including kidney damage, blindness, neuropathy, amputations, and cardiovascular disease. How have America's physicians been doing in preventing and managing this increasingly prevalent yet very manageable disease?

In the United States, DM now ranks number seven on the list of all reasons for a physician visit; and number four if pregnancies, routine checkups and other visits not involving an illness or injury are excluded. The only principal diagnoses having a higher percentage than DM of all return visits to a physician are essential hypertension (high blood pressure) and normal pregnancy. The September 1995 issue of the *Journal of the American Dietetic Association* reports that:

> Of all expenditures for diabetes, 40.5% are attributed to inpatient hospital care. This compares with 0.03% attributed to diet and nutritional counseling, and 1.0% to diagnostic testing.[5]

A study published in the April 1994 issue of the *Journal of Clinical Endocrinology and Metabolism*, which was conducted by Lewin-VHI, Inc. for the Diabetes Treatment Centers of America, estimates that costs incurred in treating people with diabetes are averaging 3.65 times more than the cost of treating the nondiabetic population. The study found that diagnosed diabetics comprise about 4.5 percent of the total population, and account for more than 15 percent of total healthcare expenditures, roughly one out of every seven dollars spent annually in the United States. The study estimates that an equivalent number of Americans may be undiagnosed diabetics, so that the expenditures on diabetes care may double within the short run. Commenting on the results of the study, Julio Pita, M.D., medical director of the Diabetes Treatment Center at Miami's Mercy Hospital, said:

> This study shows that traditional methods of treating diabetes and its complications have resulted in shockingly high health care costs. . . . We have to start treating the disease with a more aggressively preventive approach if we are to reduce the cost. . . . Because it is a chronic disease that cannot be cured, diabetes is best treated through a continuum of preventive care which keeps blood sugar levels as close to normal as possible by careful monitoring and frequent and timely use of medication. . . . This kind of preventive care with

a team of health care providers . . . can help individuals with diabetes exercise regularly, control their diets, and keep a close eye on their blood sugar levels and can help them gain greater control of their disease and suffer fewer complications. Fewer complications results in lower costs.[6]

According to a National Institutes of Health (NIH) report dated October 1995, DM is the fourth leading cause of death by disease for Americans. The NIH also found that "NIDDM (noninsulin dependent diabetes mellitus) accounts for 90 to 95 percent of diabetes."[7] The NIH estimated that direct and indirect costs of diabetes care in the United States were over $137 billion annually. The estimates are that 16 million Americans are diabetic, 8 million of them diagnosed, and 8 million undiagnosed.

As a result of the disease and its complications, people with diabetes have more frequent and intensive encounters with the health care system. . . . (People with diabetes) . . . are at increased risk of developing chronic complications related to ophthalmic, renal, neurological, cerebrovascular, cardiovascular, and peripheral vascular disease. Diabetics, for example, are more likely than their nondiabetic peers to have heart attacks, strokes, amputations, kidney failure, and blindness.[8]

This study concluded that total expenditures for direct health care of diabetics in 1992 were $102 billion, or 15 percent of total U.S. healthcare expenditures for that year. Although no more current dollar figure has yet been reported for total direct expenditures for diabetes care, the Novemebr 1997 issue of *Disease Management* confirms that these costs remain at the level of 15 percent of total U.S. healthcare expenditures. It is noteworthy that Medicare has been paying about 44 percent of these acute care costs.

Representative Elizabeth Furse (D–Oregon) introduced HR 58 on January 7, 1997, to: "help improve the quality of life for 16 million Americans who have diabetes." Her remarks on introducing this bill included the following statistics:

- Diabetes is the leading cause of kidney failure requiring dialysis— costing Medicare $1.8 billion every year.

- Diabetes is the leading cause of amputations—costing Medicare $2 billion every year. Fifty percent of these amputations are preventable.

- Ninety percent of diabetes-related blindness is preventable.

- Fifty percent of diabetes-related kidney disease is preventable.

- Fifty percent of diabetes-related hospitalizations are preventable.

- Diabetic skin ulcers are responsible for approximately 60,000 limb amputations each year. The average cost of each primary amputation is $40,500. This represents a $2.4 billion annual cost to the American healthcare system.

An epidemiologist named Maureen Harris, coeditor of *Diabetes in America*, reports that:

> The prevalence (of DM) has increased dramatically over time and is now five times the prevalence measured in 1958. Rates rise from 1.5% at age 18 to 44 years and 6.5% at age 45 to 64 years to 10–11% at ages greater than 65 years. . . . Further, about 20 million people have impaired glucose tolerance (IGT), a condition in which blood glucose levels are not diabetic but are clearly greater than normal, and which conveys high risk for heart disease and subsequent development of diabetes.[9]

Despite this dramatic increase in the prevalence of the disease, DM, and particularly NIDDM, represent very manageable diseases. Many physicians would consider them among the most manageable of the leading chronic diseases.

> The National Institutes of Health recently released the results of the 10-year Diabetes Control and Complications Trial (DCCT). It proved that aggressive control of blood sugar levels can prevent or delay the costly complications of diabetes. It shows that costs can be significantly reduced, while dramatically improving the health status of people with diabetes. To accomplish these exciting results, we not only have to do things differently, we have to do different things. We cannot treat this chronic disease with an acute intervention approach. The solution requires continuous, proactive disease management strategies that integrate the necessary services into a seamless whole.[10]

In a study of the overall effectiveness of diabetes care in the United States, epidemologist David Marrero offered the following concluding remarks:

How might we judge the quality of care being provided to people with NIDDM by primary care physicians (PCPs)? The brief overview presented here using state and national samples suggests that despite considerable efforts to disseminate practice guidelines in the last decade, there continue to be gaps between the current recommendations for care and actual PCP practices. Specifically, for patients with NIDDM, methods for assessing chronic glycemic control and strategies for the screening and treatment of retinopathy, nephropathy, and foot problems are not uniformly applied. Moreover, in most surveys, the data suggest that patients with NIDDM receive less aggressive treatment and fewer preventive services than patients with IDDM. The reasons for this finding are unknown. However, it may be inferred from the data that PCPs may perceive NIDDM as a less serious illness than IDDM. From a public health standpoint, providing fewer preventive services to people with NIDDM greatly increases the burden of diabetes, because NIDDM constitutes the majority of cases, and some complications, such as cardiovascular and foot disease, are more common in NIDDM patients.[11]

Anne L. Peters, M.D., professor of medicine in the Division of Endocrinology at UCLA's School of Medicine, wrote as follows in her 1996 commentary on a study by R. G. Hiss, R. M. Anderson, G. E. Hess, C. J. Stepien, and W. K. Davis entitled "Community Diabetes Care," published in the journal *Diabetes Care*:

Why, with the advances in technology and an increasing awareness of the value of maintaining near-euglycemia, is the quality of diabetes care so poor in almost every setting in which it is measured? Part of the problem stems from a lack of knowledge on the part of both patients and physicians regarding appropriate glycemic goals and how to achieve them. Second, while busy physicians may ask patients to collect SMBG (self-monitoring blood glucose) data, these physicians often do not act upon the data in a timely and effective fashion. Management decisions must be closely linked to the collection of SMBG and laboratory results. (Often the required laboratory tests are not obtained at all.) One example, from a chart review of patients with diabetes, is a chart on which it was noted "blood glucose level=450 mg/dl [milligrams per deciliter], continue glyburide, return to clinic 1 year."[12]

Patients with a blood glucose level of 450 mg/dl should not be permitted to leave the clinic without immediate treatment to gradually reduce their blood glucose level. It is unconscionably bad medical practice to otherwise release these patients, much less to dismiss them for an entire year.

The Diabetes Educator dated July/August 1991, reports that Pennsylvania State University researchers "surveyed over 600 primary care physicians and discovered that over 90% did not read any diabetes publications. Only 2.6% read *Diabetes Care*, the primary clinical journal of the American Diabetes Association. The care provided by the physicians was deficient in four major categories: patient use of home blood glucose monitors, frequency of glycoslyated hemoglobin measurement [a measurement of the amount of sugar attached to red blood cells], routine referrals to eye doctors, and routine foot examinations."

Each year, the eight million diagnosed diabetics account for over sixteen million physician visits, and what happens to them during those visits adds up to a very sad and enduring story of inadequate and poor quality medical performance. Diabetic patients too often leave their primary physicians' offices with no complete, accurate knowledge about their disease. Many have reported being told: "Take one of these pills daily, and don't eat sugar." Most health insurers will not pay for blood sugar monitoring equipment unless the disease has progressed to the stage of insulin dependence; and few insurers will pay for the test strips necessary in using the monitor. As a consequence of ignorance of their disease, blood-sugar levels skyrocket and plunge; many complications occur; hospitalization for "diabetes out of control" becomes a frequent occurrence; toes, feet, and legs are amputated; people lose their eyesight; and these patients suffer a much higher incidence of stroke, heart attack, and peripheral vascular problems.

The dismal record of diabetes care in America, as the twentieth century comes to a close, illustrates the point made previously that the "remainder of things" has been lost sight of by the physician, for the reason that the scheme of ideas which is now guiding physician behavior includes the consistent mistaking of the *abstract* for the concrete, which Whitehead has termed the *fallacy of misplaced concreteness,* a logical fallacy spawned by the cosmological notions of the seventeenth century. The American physician is in fact treating "an organism with a specific genetic and environmental history, having complex biochemical, physiological and psychological processes continuously going on," however his conventional medical abstractions, based as they are upon an erroneous scheme of ideas, have tended to blind him to the living, concrete realities that must certainly be dealt with as the new millennium arrives.

In the July 1996 issue of *Diabetes Care,* William W. Fore, M.D., one of twelve partners in a physician clinic, stated that:

> Many physicians "talk the talk, but they don't walk the walk." While recognizing that diabetes should be treated, that obesity should be treated, that hyperlipidemia should be treated, and so on, they find it easy to take care of diabetes during the asymptomatic period. Then they refer (the DM patient) when they're blind and nephrotic.[13]

The February 1997 issue of *Diabetes Care* quotes Raymond Fabius, Medical Director of U.S Healthcare/Aetna, as stating that 90 percent of the direct costs for nearly 40,000 diabetic members were incurred by 2,000 of those patients; and 50 percent of total costs were incurred by the 300 most ill patients. These are the disastrous wages of "talking the talk, but not walking the walk" when it comes to caring for patients who have diabetes.

How else might the quality and efficacy of diabetes care in America be judged? The World Health Organization (WHO) regularly gathers clinical data on the causes of death, based upon ICD–9 (*International Classification of Diseases,* 9th edition) disease/diagnosis codes. The WHO reports include deaths from all causes, and deaths in each specific ICD–9 category. A comparison of the incidence of deaths caused by diabetes in the United States with those in the United Kingdom over a recent five year period will provide an additional concrete and reliable basis for such judgment. The following table is based on data from the World Health Statistics Annual 1993.[14]

Year	*Country*	*Deaths/All Causes*	*Deaths/DM*	*%/Total*	*+or-*
1988	USA	2,167,999	40,368	1.8%	
1992	USA	2,185,673	50,067	2.3%	+24%
1989	UK	657,733	8,486	1.3%	
1993	UK	658,733	6,748	1.0%	-20%

In the United States, there were 17,674 more deaths from all causes in 1992 than in 1988. There were 9,699 more deaths from diabetes mellitus in 1992 than in 1988. This means that 55 percent of the *increase* in American deaths in 1992 were caused by DM. There was an *increase* of 27 percent in the rate of DM-caused deaths as a percentage of deaths from all causes. In the United Kingdom, the statistics tell a quite different story. There were 748 more deaths from all causes in 1993 as compared with 1989; and there were 1,663 fewer deaths from diabetes in 1993 than in 1989. The United Kingdom experienced a 76 percent *decrease* in the rate of DM-caused deaths as a percentage of deaths from all causes.

The NIH has recently published findings of serious underreporting of diabetes mellitus by physicians, and has suggested that the correct number of DM-caused deaths in the United States in 1992 was 169,000 or 3.4 times the number reported to the World Health Organization. The comparison of WHO data for a five year period demonstrates clearly that British physicians and their patients are managing diabetes—a very manageable disease—in a manner that yields outcomes far superior to those resulting from the medical practices of American physicians.

After a review of the foregoing facts about the management and the outcomes of diabetes care in America, and after careful consideration of such unsettling and irreducible facts revealed about American medicine and its comparative accomplishments in the contemporary world, who is likely to believe that we enjoy "the best medical care in the world"? These particulars suggest that, to the contrary, American society is being hoodwinked by the free barons of the American medical guild. The harsh truth cannot be avoided: the recent, widely praised history of medicine in the United States can also be read as a series of disastrous failures that have occurred in spite of, and in some measure because of, the generous endowment by the American people of medical education, and of medicine in most every aspect. The dismal record cited in the foregoing paragraphs with regard to diabetes mellitus is but one example of such failure.

Given the explosion of high-tech diagnostic and treatment modalities and the radical escalation in the cost of inpatient hospital care during the past thirty years, the old saying about the value of an ounce of prevention needs to be revised: an ounce of prevention would now be worth a ton of cure. The disturbing morbidity and mortality statistics cited for Americans with diabetes mellitus are the direct result of an approach to medical care that values tons of cure very highly, and that places no value whatsoever upon the ounce of prevention. Even if primary doctors had all of the information needed to effectively manage patients with NIDDM—which they clearly do not have—they would not find the time or have the inclination to teach this information to their diabetic patients. There is no reimbursement to be had for teaching patients about their disease within a fee-for-service practice, which creates an overwhelming disincentive for the physician. Judged on the basis of documented outcomes for the diabetic patient, and taking, for example, the comparison of WHO statistics on DM as a cause of death, the approach of providing tons of cure from the point at which the patient has developed serious complications from DM is very clearly not the right thing to do medically for the patient. In addition to being bad medical practice, it is also the most wasteful path for the physician to pursue in terms of the burden on society caused by the extraordinary cost to be borne as the direct result of a "tons of cure" approach to this chronic, yet manageable illness. Who benefits from this wrongheaded approach? No one—absolutely no one—other than the physicians involved and the parts of the medical establishment that support their inappropriate activities.

Public Health and Private Medicine

Improvements achieved in the health status of Americans are the result of policies, discoveries, and interventions in the arena of public health that have dramatically reduced, and in some cases eliminated, diseases and threats to health that were causing a great deal of morbidity and mortality. Population-based interventions, especially during the first half of the twentieth century, have produced most of the statistical improvements in the health status of American citizens. There is no evidence that the practices of private physicians in their private offices and hospital workshops have had any positive impact on the statistics that provide a measure of the health status of the population. The statistics for deaths caused by DM will suffice to buttress this conclusion. American society has plainly misunderstood these facts, and it has given credence to the constant claims by the AMA and the medical guild that practicing physicians deserve the credit for improvements in health status indicators, which have been achieved chiefly through the population-based medicine of public health physicians, nurses, and laboratory scientists. The Pew Health Professions Commission offers this perspective:

While our nation's huge investment in biomedical research has paid dividends, they are not equal, by a factor of five, to the gains in life expectancy owed to changes in nutrition, sanitation, prevention, and other public health measures. Attention to population-based approaches to health care will have to become better balanced with biomedical approaches. Focusing attention on the health status of individuals and communities will be the key to realizing this balance.[15]

Primary Care Is Primary

Returning to the discussion of the need for a "reversal of centers" in medical education and in medical practice in the United States, the center of the medical cosmos needs to be surrendered to (some would say *returned* to) the generalist physician, to doctors trained in primary care and in family medicine, whose training has taken place within a radically altered scheme and setting for medical education. Ian McWhinney, M.D., who has dedicated his professional life as a teacher and practitioner to the propagation of this gospel, has made the following observations:

> The Flexner reforms prepared the way for medicine to become a technology. As in so many other areas of modern life, however, the benefits of technology have been reaped without steps taken to contain and control its negative effects. . . . Among the most serious problems thrown up by the [Flexner] reforms . . . that of primary care . . . has been identified by many writers as the central issue: . . . the question of who should be the doctor of first contact. . . . In the university center, the demands of academic life—of teaching, research, and administration—are often in conflict with the task of being a family doctor. . . . Primacy of the person may be incompatible with the primacy of publication. . . . To restore the primacy of the person, one needs a medicine that puts the person in all his wholeness in the center of the stage and does not separate the disease from the man, and the man from his environment—a medicine that makes technology firmly subservient to human values, and maintains a creative balance between generalist and specialist. These I believe to be the aims of family medicine. . . . [The] crucial issue [is]: the question whether physicians are prepared to put their commitment to people above their commitment to technology. . . . [T]he kind of commitment I am speaking of implies that the physician

will "stay with" a person whatever his problem may be, and he will do so because his commitment is to people more than to a body of knowledge or a branch of technology. . . . It is a . . . distortion of reality to talk as if people's problems are neatly divided into "organic" and "psychosocial" categories. People are ill as wholes not as parts. . . . Learning to be a family physician requires a change of perspective that can only take place where the new perspective is dominant. It will . . . be apparent why I think that attempts to produce a family doctor by putting together a conventional training in pediatrics and internal medicine—and adding some psychiatry—are doomed to failure. "The whole is different from the sum of its parts." Family doctors may emerge in this way, but they will do so by the arduous route of rising above their training and learning from their own experience. . . . Family physicians have in common the fact that they obtain fulfillment from personal relations more than from the technical aspects of medicine. Their commitment is to a group of people more than to a body of knowledge. Their experience gives them a distinctive perspective of illness that includes its personal and social context.[16]

The commitment, for the teacher and for the learner, must also be to the *management of a process of care* in contrast to the prevalent focus on *treatment of an episode of illness*. A 1995 Pew Health Professions Commission report that is loaded with important insights into the flaws of the present healthcare system includes the following observations:

The system is oriented to serving individuals and their immediate treatment needs and not to recognizing disease and disability as products of multiple influences: psychological, social, behavioral, economic, and political. . . . [T]he American health care system, without the benefit of a capacity for self-correction, has grown to the point where it endangers public and private spending on other essential activities. In the face of this unsustainable growth a frightening reality confronts the American public: . . . the largest cohort in the nation's history, the Baby Boom generation, does not turn 60 until 2006. When this cohort reaches retirement, it will place even more strain on a system which is failing today.[17]

In this failing system, operating as it is "without the benefit of a capacity for self-correction," the need to reverse the centers in medical education and in the hierarchy of medicine has become an inescapable necessity, in part because medicine is functioning today without the benefit of a general manager. Unless a way can be found to rapidly reverse the present pattern, and to reconstruct the scheme of ideas along distinctly different lines, solidly resituating the generalist physician at the center of the medical cosmos, the eventual collapse of American medicine will be inevitable. The Pew Health Professions Commission has offered the following in one of its reports:

> During the last century, the U.S. medical profession has been transformed from a system dominated by general practitioners into a body of highly specialized physicians. In 1931, more than four out of five physicians (80%) were in general practice, yet after World War II, the proportion of physicians who were generalists fell rapidly. By 1965 the proportion dropped to about one-half (50%), and by 1990, the percentage of physicians in generalist areas had decreased to approximately one-third (33%) of all physicians. In most Western nations, the percentage of primary care physicians far exceeds that of the United States, with 50% of Canadian physicians and 70% of the British as general practice or family physicians . . . [S]ome studies indicate that the relative emphasis on specialized services in the United States does not result in improvements in broad measures of health status.[18]

The crisis that threatened to destroy the Chrysler Corporation some years ago provides a fitting analogy. If left to the free barons of American medicine to resolve the financial and organizational crises faced by the automaker, instead of nominating a high-paid fellow like Lee Iacocca as the new general manager, and giving him the resources and the authority to reconstruct the company, the American medical guild would have pursued its own unique formula for success:

- Eliminate the expense of a general manager as unnecessary.

- Rely on specialists in each aspect of design, manufacture, and sales to operate the company. Being specialists they can do it better.

- Any generalists who are employed must be placed in the most labor-intensive, lowest-paid positions, and must be constantly reminded that they belong right where they are, at the very bottom of the totem.

The scheme of ideas would be simple: by relying on its experts in instrumentation, frames, metallurgy, drive trains, wheels, tires, fabric, paints, electronics, trim, robotics, production, purchasing, warehousing, distribution, shipping and transportation, and marketing, fabulous automobiles would be produced without the need for general management. Everyone would do their own specific part of the job expertly; everyone would keep their own records systems, and share as little information as possible; and coordination of these diverse and various individual efforts would occur automatically. Chrysler would have made a miraculous recovery without Lee Iacocca, or someone like him, because the need for a general manager to bring order out of chaos in a complex human endeavor did not exist. All it would take is specialists, and lots and lots of them. Cost, quite naturally, would not be a consideration. After all, when the focus is on quality, one should never concern oneself about price.

The foregoing may be perceived as mere sarcasm; however, this is a fair description of the precise situation that exists in fee-for-service medicine in America today. There is no general medical manager, despite claims to the contrary; there is no systematic clinical evaluation, and therefore no assurance of quality; and the society has been paying an enormous and radically increasing price—in money and in relative health status—because of these glaring defects. Medicine cannot progress as a true science unless it recognizes the need to resituate its generalist physicians in a central role, as the key managers of the processes of care for patients with chronic and acute problems, and as effective agents in the promotion of health.

Achieving a "reversal of centers" in academic medicine and in the field of medical practice will prove to be extremely difficult. Physician free barons, particularly those in academia, are not likely to surrender any part of their present power, status, influence, or income on a voluntary basis, much less as the result of a reawakening of Hippocratic zeal. In their December 1995 report entitled *Critical Challenges: Revitalizing the Health Professions for the Twenty-First Century,* the PEW Health Professions Commission said:

> The difficulty of changing the established patterns of professional education and practice should not be underestimated. . . . For instance, while there is little doubt that medical specialties are in oversupply, the government still subsidizes graduate medical education with over $6.5 billion

annually, most of which goes to train more specialists. . . . The subsidy for
education that is tied to care delivery must be broken. . . . To address the
changes in health in a responsive manner will require the bold action of
leaders in all sectors of the system. Bold action is not something that has
typified the governance of the profession or, for that matter, higher education. Like so much of today's health care system, this attitude must change.
Fundamental alterations in the processes that govern professional education, regulate the professions, orient professions to practice and finance
education will be required. This will mean action at the federal, state, institutional and professional levels. . . . Professional training and practice
should place more emphasis on developing the qualities of a superb generalist, capable of comprehensive management of care, as opposed to the current orientation toward specialization. . . . The current environment of
overspecialization, orientation toward high technology medicine, and preference for institutionally based education is the result of over 40 years of
direct and indirect federal policies. *Only a purposeful reformation of these policies will bring significant change.*[19] (Emphasis added)

It is most likely that a new "Flexner Report," backed up with the teeth
necessary to enforce implementation, will be required to bring about the
changes without which American medical care continues to mill about,
misses its opportunities for reconstruction, and eventually crashes and burns.
There is every likelihood, of course, that the outcome of forced changes for
practicing physicians will be far less acceptable to the medical profession
than the outcomes that could result from a trenchant self-analysis, and from
a self-initiated reconstruction of the scheme of ideas governing academic
medicine today, and dictating the on-line functioning of contemporary
American medicine.

In April 1994 the Pew Health Professions Commission published its
Commission Policy Papers, which would provide a decent starting point for the
development of a new "Flexner Report." Following is a sample of the Commission's findings and recommendations:

Nationally the current medical care system supports a workforce dominated by medical specialists. A reformed system should strive to . . .
"manage" patient care better. Any managed system will require a greatly
expanded primary care orientation and workforce, including family physi-

cians, general pediatricians, general internists, nurse practitioners, physician assistants, and certified nurse midwives. . . . Much of the evidence for the advantages of a primary care-based system have come from small studies and international comparisons. Its success has been exhibited in many other countries and most recently in a cross national study among seven major industrialized nations (Starfield, 1991).[20] A consensus has emerged from these studies that such a system would contribute significantly to reduced costs, expanded access, and improved quality of care. . . . Increasing the primary care workforce in the United States requires breaking tradition with the past policies that have shaped health care and professional education.

Create an appropriately sized physician workforce that is characterized by at least 50% primary care physicians and that trains each physician with the skills necessary to practice in a dramatically changed health care system.

Link . . . federal graduate medical education funding to the health care needs of the public.

Close the compensation gap between generalist and specialist physicians.

Reconstruct the system of federal support for graduate medical education to secure an adequately sized and appropriately trained primary care physician workforce.

Encourage medical schools, teaching hospitals and other health care delivery systems to develop retraining programs for equipping specialists with generalist skills.

Create public-private partnerships to facilitate state-based planning for health professional education reform.[21]

Evidence of the "chilly climate" academic medicine offers primary care at the present time suggests that restoring the generalist to a central position in the teaching of medicine, in the practice of medicine, and in the regulation of both, will have to be forced upon the American medical guild. Given all the indicators that the free barons leading the American medical guild lack the capacity to evaluate and correct the erroneous scheme of ideas that propels them today, it would be naive to expect those in power to turn the current medical totem on its head, shove the surgical "top guns" from the center of the medical cosmos, and turn the central role and real power over to the very same generalist physicians whose welcome in academia is described as "chilly." It appears certain that the required reversal of centers will have to be accomplished by the use of brute political and economic power. Otherwise it will not occur, and the progression to eventual disaster will continue unabashed. The kind of clout that Abraham Flexner wielded in 1910 will have to be mustered again in order to achieve a true reorientation of medical education, and a thoroughgoing reconstruction of medical practice. The leverage of $12.6 billion in annual state and federal subsidies for medical education and research can be used to encourage the free barons to learn how to resituate generalist physicians as the genuine center and directional force of a new medical cosmos.

A "reversal of centers" must begin with radical change in the criteria for selecting medical students. Forty-five thousand men and women apply for admission to medical schools each year in the hope of filling approximately 16,000 places. The number of slots will have to be sharply decreased for a period of years to assist in reducing the current oversupply of physicians; thus medical schools must become even more selective. Selection criteria must be reoriented toward breadth of intelligence and knowledge; subtlety and openness of mind; interpersonal reverence and high placement on the "socioemotional" index; organizing, integrating, and managing abilities; a keen interest in and commitment to primary medical care and family medicine; and what Ian McWhinney has termed "insight and awareness . . . an integral part of the personality." Selection criteria must be reoriented to avoid the impression that a higher value is placed on memory than on insight and awareness; or that a warm welcome is given to those who exhibit narrow technical interests and a focus on specialized knowledge, while students with more general interests and a high placement on the so-called socioemotional index experience a "chilly" reception; or that greater respect is paid to students with a high interest in earning the big dollars, and a corollary disrespect is shown for anyone interested in a career in primary care. The reconstructed selection criteria should also implicitly recognize surgeons for what they are: glorified mechanics.

At least 50 percent of all medical school openings must be in primary care: family medicine, general pediatrics, and general internal medicine; and the climate for generalism must shift from "chilly" to very comfortable.

Training at both the undergraduate and graduate levels must be radically altered to include the siting of at least 50 percent of clinical experience in ambulatory care settings away from the academic center and in the community, preferably within the clinical centers of well-run "managed-care" or HMO organizations. Curricula must be revised to reflect an understanding that care giving involves a long-term process, not an episode. Physicians must be trained to manage a longitudinal process of care, and to recognize that, as with every other human enterprise, the general manager (in this case the generalist physician) is the central actor in assuring that an optimal outcome will result from the process of care.

In the world outside of contemporary American medicine there is no doubt that the general manager is the key to corporate success, which is why general managers usually receive the highest financial rewards. This notion is clearly at odds with the scheme of ideas underlying the behavior of America's physician free barons. The prevailing categories of importance assigned to the various "specialties" within medicine must change, as well as the relative distribution of economic rewards among these professional categories. The general medical manager must be appropriately compensated.

Reconstruction along these lines, with the generalist physician firmly placed in a central position, would make it possible to overcome the bifurcation of "basic science" and "clinical medicine" which has undermined medical inquiry during most of the twentieth century. As Ian McWhinney has observed:

> It would be impossible to apply advances in basic science without a body of scientific knowledge which is only obtainable from clinical observation. In the study of human illness, the ultimate test of any chemical or physical analysis must be: what are its implications for the survival and functioning of the whole organism? And this is a question which can only be answered by clinical observation. . . . Clinical observation, then, is not only a scientific discipline, but it is *the* science of medicine. . . . Clinical medicine . . . is an observational science. It is one of those sciences which, in Ryle's words, tries to "establish the truth of things by observing and recording, by classification and analysis."[22]

In April 1996, Dr. Ian McWhinney delivered the William Pickles Lecture at the spring meeting of the Royal College of General Practitioners in

Aberdeen, Scotland. His lecture was titled "The Importance of Being Different." (The lecture was subsequently published in the July 1996 edition of the *British Journal of General Practice.*) McWhinney identified four principal characteristics which differentiate medical generalists from medical "specialists," and which distinguish primary care from all other medical disciplines:

1. "It is the only discipline to define itself in terms of relationships, especially the doctor-patient relationship."

2. "General practitioners tend to think in terms of individual patients rather than generalized abstractions."

3. "General practice is based on an organismic rather than a mechanistic metaphor of biology."

4. "General practice is the only major field which transcends the dualistic division between mind and body."

Dr. McWhinney's lecture concluded with the following words:

The four differences I have described are all of a piece. Giving primacy to long-term relationships directs our attention to the particulars of illness; and the complexity of illness in the context of relationships makes it difficult for us to think in mechanistic and dualistic terms. But we have hardly begun to see the advantages of our position. Transcending the "fault line" should make general practice the ideal therapeutic setting for the many disorders which, like chronic pain, do not fit neatly on one side or the other. The more we learn about the effect of supportive relationships on cancer and other chronic diseases, the more redundant the fault line becomes. To realize our potential, however, we have other work to do. Thinking in the way I have described may be natural for us, but it is still difficult, for we are all, to some extent, prisoners of an unreformed clinical method and the language of linear causation and mind/body dualism. The fault line runs through the affect-denying clinical method which dominates the modern medical school. Not until this is reformed will emotions and relationships have the place in medicine they deserve. Finally, to become self-reflective, medicine will have to go through a huge cultural change. In these changes, general practice is already some distance along the way. The importance of being different is that we can lead the way.[23]

The message that the medical profession has gotten itself into deep trouble by its failure to understand and appreciate the *difference* about the family physician, and by its persistent negligence of the *importance* of this difference could hardly be stated better than Dr. McWhinney has done.

Reorganizing Medical Information

The second aspect of the thoroughgoing reconstruction of American medicine is the need for a reconstruction of medical information. If a contest was held today among the major enterprises in society to select the one with the worst approach to capturing, recording, organizing, protecting, using, reporting and managing information, it is indisputable that medicine would win the prize, hands down. American physicians take a perverse sort of pride in the fact that no one can read their handwriting except themselves. There are cases on record indicating that, during external auditing of medical charts by regulatory or legal authorities, physicians in some instances have admitted that they were unable to decipher their own scrawlings. Two hallmarks of the medieval guild were the solemn commitment to secrecy, and the use of a secret language to restrict the flow of certain information exclusively to guild members. These commitments were an important element in the feudal compact, and were reflected in the procedures by which free barons protected their turf. The American medical guild has long maintained an analogous interest in insuring that the information entered into a medical chart is the property of the physician writing it down, and not available to any other person without the express concurrence of the author. Not even the patient may see this information. Physicians have relied on Latin shorthand to insure secrecy for some record entries.

As a result of these patterns and procedures, medical record shelves in private physician offices throughout the country are filled with patient files containing information inaccessible for the most fundamental purposes of *the* science of medicine: the systematic recording of clinical observations for a defined patient population as a source for continuously evaluating the health status of that patient population, and of assessing the performance of the physician in managing the medical problems patients present.

The Organization of Clinical Information

More than two decades ago, Peter Drucker predicted that the dynamic force that would characterize the twenty-first century, much as "scientific revolution" and "industrial revolution" have marked the preceding centuries, would be the information revolution. His precise words were "the organization of information." As has always been the case, new centuries have a way of leaping over the precise numerical boundaries we set for them: the world is already well into an information revolution, and therefore in some ways already into the dynamics of the twenty-first century. No segment of American culture stands more in need of a reconstruction of its approaches to gathering and managing information than does the medical-care system.

In undertaking the reconstruction and reorganization of medicine's approach to information, the most significant fact to which attention must be paid is that the core of medicine, the central event around which all else rotates, is the encounter of the patient with the primary-care physician. Anyone who argues or believes otherwise has things backward. The importance of capturing the information and data from these encounters must not be underestimated. Here is the source of continuously reconsidering and reconstructing the abstractions that drive and influence the practicing physician; and here is the source of an ongoing revision of the classifications that guide and often control medical practice. Here is the source of creating rational places to put the results of significant clinical observations which, at a given moment, may not fit within the ordained set of medical classifications. Here is the source of information that can lead to the promulgation of new, practical, and realistic guidelines for those illnesses seen most frequently by the primary physician; and for those illnesses that present the greatest challenges in terms of managing the processes of care. Here also is the principal source of the scientific information, rooted in broad clinical experience, that will be required if the patterns of medical education and the topics of medical research are to be successfully reconstructed, as a corollary of a "reversal of centers" in the academy. What will be required is a clear recognition that the collective clinical experience of generalist physicians in the primary-care setting, and the diligent recording of their clinical observations, constitutes *the* true science of medicine, offering the only practical and realistic means of achieving coherence and continuity across the fields of medical education, research, and practice.

Accomplishing an information revolution in medicine presents enormous challenges. The first thing for the medical guild is to recognize that its "secret language" approach must be abandoned, and that the new medical information system must be an open system. That is, information from clinical observation must be captured in a form that will facilitate working with the information and using it to construct epidemiological and statistical databases for evaluating the nature of the "risks" in the patient population, and for analyzing variations in practice patterns that may suggest inappropriate or excessive care.

Accomplishing an information revolution in medicine along the foregoing lines will require the routine capture of primary-care clinical observations in a machine-readable form, using a language that will facilitate accurate understanding of the meaning of the information being put into the computer. The challenge of arriving at a unified, machine-intelligent medical language is a complex but centrally important one for the profession. The great promise of such a revolution in medical information cannot be fulfilled unless physicians learn how to provide machine-ready data for input into the computer, so that the machine can do its work and the information can then be queried and put to practical use as the principal basis for an ongoing evaluative clinical science. American medicine has so far largely avoided the crucial issue of how to put medical information into the computer in a way that the computer can recognize and handle.

Self-Help in Primary Care

Given the hectic and time-constrained nature of primary-care practice today, how will it be possible for these busy physicians to handle the added burdens of an information revolution? One response to this significant question can be found in a retrospective look at the retail grocery business. Prior to World War II, in major metropolitan areas of this country, the "supermarket" had not yet emerged, and competing grocery retailers were often located in much smaller quarters. They would gladly accept telephone orders from customers, assemble and package the order, and dispatch an "order boy" with a pushcart to deliver the goods to the customer's home. The groceries would be carried into the kitchen; the payment due would be collected; and the order boy would walk his empty cart back to the store. Just imagine what a loaf of bread or a quart of milk would cost today if this approach to delivering groceries to consumers had persisted until now. Few would be able to afford the luxury of groceries. The reconstruction of the retail grocery business has been accomplished through the supermarket, and the central change has been that customers are required to do more for themselves. Customers must travel to and from the store; they must select the merchandise from the shelves, place the goods on the cashier's counter; perhaps help in bagging the groceries; pay for them on the spot; and carry them to the car and home.

An analogous sort of reconstruction must occur in medical care: patients must be required to do more for themselves. Based upon currently existing technology, for example, instead of having patients sit passively for a period of time in the primary physician's waiting room, the site can be equipped to enable patients to record their own height, weight, pulse, heart rate, temperature, blood pressure, blood glucose, lung capacity, balance, and muscle strength. For each individual patient who performs these self-tests, the physician can be provided with an immediate on-screen report or with a printout of the results. No nurse time and no physician time would be required to make this useful and timely data available for the physician. Such data would cumulatively form a very significant part of the patient's medical history, in electronic and machine-readable form.

Another response to the question of how a busy primary-care physician can handle the added burdens of an information revolution can be found by examining the data-management resources currently in use in large and busy restaurants. The key to rapid data entry to facilitate communication between waiters and cooks is the touch screen, using a series of templates pertinent to the food-service business. In medicine, the template for "sore throat" could be selected with a touch or two on the computer screen, and the physician could then go in and enter or edit information for the specific patient and medical problem at hand.

Changing Medicine's "Natural" Language

In order to realize these prospects, there will have to be a parsing of current medical language on a system-wide basis. That is, the "natural" language of medical science must be analyzed and reformed into a unified medical language that can be easily captured in electronic form, and made usable by the machine for the pivotal purposes of supporting clinical performance as well as for subsequent clinical evaluation and relevant research. The parsing of current medical language is of central importance in developing a user-friendly system of rapid data entry that does not require a "computer nerd" to make effective use of the templates or to realize the direct clinical benefits to be gained from the outputs of the computerized information system. Each and every practicing physician must become comfortable with a reformed medical language and with the new machine tools, and receive the training necessary in order to achieve a high comfort level for themselves. More importantly, each and every physician must be easily able to recognize the value that the reorganized clinical information can provide to enhance the management of the processes of care required by patients.

Voice technology, currently in use in efficient radiology practices and in emergency medicine, also holds significant promise for enhancing the ability of primary-care physicians to more efficiently capture clinical data in electronic form. This technology needs to be stretched to a more practical fit with the requirements of primary-care medicine.

Aside from the parsing of traditional medical language, there is the challenging issue of reorganizing the general structure of medical information to reflect a "reversal of centers," i.e., to give full recognition to the central position of the primary physician at the heart of *the* science of medicine—clinical observation at the point of first contact. The traditional principle of organizing medical information has been to record data based upon the source of medical care. Within an academic medical center, for example, the ob/gyn clinic would keep records on the progress of a pregnancy, including notation of a patient referral to the cardiology clinic located down the hall when a slight heart murmur has been detected. The cardiology clinic would establish its own medical record for the referred patient, and independently diagnose and treat the patient. Because there has traditionally been no practical means to relate the decisions and actions of one clinic to another operating within the same "center of excellence," it has been quite possible for the cardiologist to prescribe to a referred patient a medication that would be contraindicated if there was knowledge of a medication that the ob/gyn had prescribed for the same patient. Unless the patient spoke up, the contraindication could easily be missed. Another example from the real world of academic "centers of excellence" involves a teenaged patient with an undersized liver and marginal liver function, who had been a regular on the "medicine" floor for nine months, most often on a short-stay or outpatient basis, and who was a potential candidate for a liver transplant. During a weekend, this young woman had a critical episode and was taken to the medical center's emergency room by relatives. A decision was made to admit her, and she was sent to the "surgery" floor. This patient's medical history was located within the building, but on a different floor than surgery, in a different department, with no clear or straightforward means of record access across those boundaries. Despite the patient having informed the surgical residents that her body could not handle a normal level of fluids, the decision was made to insert an IV to maintain hydration at a normal level. This treatment resulted in the condition known as ascites, which is an "abnormal accumulation of serous fluid in the peritoneal cavity," and, within twenty-four hours, the young woman was dead. Physician review of this death concluded that, had the decision been made to admit her to the "medicine" floor; or had there been a ready means of obtaining the record of the ongoing treatment of this patient within another department of the "center of excellence," the surgical residents would undoubtedly not have made the same decision, and the young woman would undoubtedly not have died as the result of the treatment she received in that university medical center.

Gathering and recording clinical information on the basis of the *source of the care* can lead to outcomes of the kind described above: one part of the total clinical information about a given patient cannot easily be related to all other parts of the total available information in a timely fashion. This can clearly be harmful to human health, and, as we have just seen, it can even be fatal.

Computer technology provides the optimal avenue of resolution for this serious dilemma, however it is not a matter of simply acquiring a lot of expensive hardware and software. What is required to alter these patterns of practice involves changes in ways of thinking and behaving. There are new systems now in place in some parts of the country that can help address both aspects of the problem. One such system is the Problem-Oriented Medical Record (POMR), which centers the collection of all clinical information around the patient and the medical problems the patient presents.

With a general medical manager playing a central role in a reconstructed medical cosmos, some variation of the POMR will be an essential element in the effective reorganization of clinical information. Here again, a "reversal of centers" would be accomplished: instead of being centered on the *source of care,* the recording of clinical observation is centered on the medical problems presented. The resulting change in the organization of information is profound, and opens pathways to stringent evaluative clinical science, and thus to the enhancement of clinical outcomes for patients. A wholesale reorganization of clinical information along the foregoing lines, with the generalist physician in the central position, will result in the progressive rooting out of radical and inappropriate medical practices, and will lead to the restoration of medical conservatism to its traditional, and rightful, position of importance and influence as a driving force of a system of care in which Hippocrates would justifiably take pride. However, there is a long and tortuous road to be traveled by America's physician free barons before this end can be fully realized.

Reorganizing Membership Plans

Membership is the cardinal feature of an HMO that most directly results in the successful undermining of four of the five "Guild Free Choice" principles. Alain Enthoven, an economist who is Marriner S. Eccles Professor of Public and Private Management at Stanford University and who initiated the "managed competition" approach to health reform, cites a 1984 *Iowa Law Review* article by Charles D. Weller entitled "Free Choice as a Restraint of Trade in American Health Care Delivery and Insurance" as the source of his definition of "Guild Free Choice":

> The principles of this ["guild free choice"] system and their economic consequences are as follows: (1) free choice of doctor by the patient, which means that the insurer has no bargaining power with the doctor; (2) free

choice of prescription by the doctor, which prevents the insurer from applying quality assurance of appropriateness; (3) direct negotiation between doctor and patient regarding fees, which excludes the third-party payer, who would be likely to have information, bargaining power, and an incentive to negotiate to hold down fees; (4) fee-for-service payment, which allows physicians maximum control over their incomes by increasing the services provided; and (5) solo practice, because multispecialty group practice constitutes a break in the seamless web of mutual coercion through control of referrals that the medical profession has used to enforce the guild system.[24]

The four "guild free choice" principles that are immediately undermined when membership in an organized, direct-service system occurs are:

- Absolute free choice of physician,

- Fee-for-service payment by patients,

- Direct negotiation of fees with the patient,

- Solo practice.

Membership "reverses the center" of the physician-patient relationship. The concept is that primary physicians participating in the care of HMO members will know at each juncture exactly which persons fall under their responsibility as primary doctors. Once there is membership in a direct-service plan, clarity regarding longitudinal physician responsibility for patients becomes possible. The patient becomes central for the organization and for the providing of medical care.

Membership makes it possible to plan a system of direct medical services that will have the resources and the capability to effectively meet all of the medical and hospital-care needs of those enrolled in the plan, that is, the needs of a clearly defined population of patients. Membership results in feedback. In the fee-for-service system, patients who simply vote with their feet and disappear into the mist cannot and do not provide feedback. Membership eliminates any need for fee negotiation between physician and patient, except for the rare instance when a treatment at issue is not a covered plan benefit.

The extensive efforts by the AMA and its allies (noted in chapter 4) to employ anecdotal horror stories in order to convince the society that these instances are frequent, and not rare, is totally belied by the constancy of positive feelings about their HMO revealed in periodic member satisfaction surveys from around the country. In most cases, the samplings of member opinion are conducted on a sound basis, consistent with the principles of valid opinion research studies. The consistent outcome of these surveys has been scores for "satisfied" or "very satisfied" above the 90th percentile, and with results frequently in the very high 90s for questions about how satisfied the member is with their primary-care physician. Unless disputes over covered services were in fact rare occurrences, opinion survey results of so consistently positive a nature would certainly be rare. The fact is that they are quite usual, and very widespread.

In the light of the concrete advantages that the reality of membership can bring to the healthcare system, perhaps the ideal reconstruction to be advocated today would be to insure that every American has the opportunity to become a member of a fully accredited, fully qualified direct-service health plan. The fact that an estimated forty to forty-five million people in the United States have no health insurance, and have no established relationship with the medical-care system, constitutes a continuous element of instability and disequilibrium. If the entire population, including those presently uninsured, could choose enrollment in any one of various competent HMO-type health plans, the economies that would flow directly from that achievement could be utilized to cover a significant part of the cost of insuring those who are unable to pay the full cost of HMO membership on their own. Assume that twenty-five major HMOs had enrolled an average of ten million members, and that virtually everyone in the nation was therefore covered by a broad set of health benefits: an immediate result would be the *de facto* end of the physician oversupply problem, and therefore of the radical expenditure levels that have been caused by that oversupply. The dramatic reduction in the rate of increase in the cost of health insurance, which has been achieved by large employers during the past few years, gained chiefly through moving their investments in employee health insurance from indemnity insurers to HMOs, would be experienced for the population as a whole. There can be no doubt that some medical practices would close, most likely single specialty practices, and not primary care or multispecialty group practices. Economic pain would be felt as a corollary of addressing the current physician glut in

America in this manner. This pain would be the result of the market forces generated by the stratagem of enrolling the entire population within well-organized, prepaid systems of care that would have markedly different incentives than fee-based medicine, in financial terms as well as in terms of clinical performance.

Underuse and Overuse

The principal concern being expressed about HMOs has been the potential for underutilization, which is inherent in prepaid, per capita payment arrangements. Will the members of an HMO be denied needed care for economic reasons, because administrators or physicians are focused on bottom-line profits? Another "reversal of centers" is inherent in this issue: the clear economic incentive driving fee-for-service physicians is that the less you do to or for the patient, the less money you make; and the more you do to or for the patient, the more money you make. Within a system based on prepayment on a per capita or case-rate basis, an opposite incentive may indeed surface: less care may mean retention of more income, and more care may mean retention of less income.

The fundamental motivation underlying per capita prepayment, however, has been to completely remove the question of physician income from the medical encounter. If the monetary compensation needs of the physician can be met without basing that compensation on the number or the kind of services rendered to the patient, then the clear and present danger that excessive and unnecessary medical service will be provided can be eliminated. As a very thoughtful and perceptive pediatrician once said to me: "I suppose with capitation the thing is, if it is enough, it's enough." Under a prepayment scheme for the care of an enrolled population of patients over a sustained time period, the predominant motivation ought to be to maintain every patient in optimal health so that the demand for prepaid services will be held to a minimum. The healthier the patients, the less the physician workload, and since physician income is a constant, not a variable, healthy patients are a distinct value for the primary doctor.

It may be argued that HMOs have given physicians financial incentives for holding down the number of procedures or tests ordered, an approach that would reduce expense for the HMO, and provide physicians with opportunities to increase their income. Of far greater financial benefit to an HMO is a large and stable membership, satisfied with the care they receive. Losing members and having to replace them with new members is a very costly endeavor for any membership organization, and HMOs are no exception. There may be a plan here or there that shoots for the short-term gain of reducing its expenses by giving its doctors a bonus to order fewer tests or procedures, however they thereby embark on a slippery pathway leading straight to doom. There are legitimate reasons for well-run HMOs to monitor the use of certain procedures which are known to have been used inappropriately by physicians, such as unnecessary tonsillectomies and hysterectomies. Dr. Milton Roemer, the creator of "Roemer's Law" about the impact of hospital bed increases on utilization of those beds, has made the following observations about the results of the famous "strike" by physicians in Los Angeles County in 1976, protesting sudden, large increases in medical malpractice insurance premiums in California:

> [T]he withholding of elective surgery . . . was associated with a significant reduction in the county's overall mortality experience, compared with the previous five years. . . . There was a virtually steady decline of deaths during the slowdown—and as soon as the work action ended and elective surgeries resumed, there was a substantial jump in the mortality rate. These statistics lend support to the mounting evidence that people might benefit if less elective surgery were performed in the United States. . . . [M]uch elective surgery performed in the United States is of questionable value . . . greater restraint in the performance of elective surgical operations might well improve U.S. life expectancy.[25]

HMO practicing physicians should certainly make every reasonable effort to eliminate the *overutilization* of medical or surgical procedures, in the interest of insuring optimal health for their patients. The danger of an *underutilization* of medical resources does exist, and such practices as cash incentives for physicians to inappropriately withhold a test or procedure should be outlawed. The fact remains, however, that in the per capita, prepayment systems, the overriding incentive for the physicians is to do for each patient the right thing, in the right way, at the right time, using the right resources, with the decisions being guided by what is medically necessary and appropriate for the individual patient. There is no more quality-efficient, cost-effective approach for HMOs interested in long-term business survival, and in the continuous well being of their members who require medical care.

Nonetheless, this ideal of optimal health in the membership and of minimal demand on the physician has not been easy to achieve in medical care. Reasonable safeguards against the temptation by physicians or health-plan administrators to withhold needed services so as to maximize profits are clearly required. Because of the fact of membership, these safeguards are also immediately available. First, under the scenario of twenty-five HMO plans having divided the entire population among them through competitive marketing of their benefits, a major bottom-line goal would inevitably be retention of those members, since turnover is very costly. Each time a member leaves, that person must be replaced to maintain a stable business, and replacement would mean convincing people to switch from their present plan, and join a different plan. These efforts at retention and attracting new members cost money that would not need to be spent if the members can be retained. Once this longitudinal interest is well established within an HMO, the incentive in providing medical care focuses on doing for each patient the right thing, at the right time, in the right way, using the right resources: the four Rs. Any different behavior by plan physicians or administrators would constitute a waste of time and money. The fundamental theory underlying the per capita prepayment approach is that optimal health in the membership is profitable for the HMO, and poor health is not profitable.

Second, the presence of rip-off artists in the nation, some of them in the healthcare business, must be paid due attention, and protective procedures therefore must be in place. Here again, the fact of membership, in combination with the presence of an information system organized so as to meet Drucker's notion of a twenty-first century *information revolution,* will produce the required protections.

The True Measure of Value for Money

There are medical-care information systems already in the market with the capacity to produce population-based reports for use in the continuous monitoring and evaluation of physician performance, as well as the performance of other clinical, institutional, and administrative components of the medical-care delivery system. One such product is the Pandora MCIS, a software system owned by the Codman Research Group of New Hampshire, founded by Drs. John Wennberg and Philip Caper. This system has been designed to extract enrollment/population, claims/cost, and clinical/provider information contained in an HMO's data-management system, and to download these data to a server that can then produce a broad set of reports in graphic and tabular form for physicians and other managers to use in monitoring, profiling, and evaluating the performance of the medical-care delivery system. To quote a Pandora brochure:

> *Pandora* converts large volumes of raw health claims data into population-based health care information displays and reports customized to your specific needs. In addition, *Pandora* lets you compare your own data with similar pre-existing data from other populations. . . . We maintain the most comprehensive database on hospital in-patient care in the country. . . . This includes over 65 percent of all hospital discharges in the U.S. and 100 percent of Medicare enrollees.

This latter feature provides the basis for a "severity" or "morbidity" adjuster to be used by the HMO in evaluating its own experience, taking into account differences between the broad national database and the characteristics of its own membership in terms of gender, age, morbidity, or other factors that influence utilization patterns, and therefore costs. This system has the capacity, given the required inputs, to report on the management of all patients diagnosed with NIDDM, for example—to clearly illustrate how well these patients are being managed. How many newly diagnosed patients have been referred to a diabetes educator to learn about their disease, and about how best to manage it? How many have been provided with a glucose monitor, and a prescription for a sufficient quantity of test strips to use the monitor at least twice each day? What has been the average number of post-diagnosis physician visits for these patients? Have their extremities been appropriately examined during the visits? Have the patients been counseled on the importance of weight loss and regular exercise? (Ninety percent of NIDDM patients are obese.) How many have been to an emergency room or hospitalized for "diabetes out of control"? How many have had toes, feet, or legs amputated?

These reports can reflect the entire population of HMO members with a diagnosis of NIDDM; or compare the NIDDM members who use a specific physician or clinic with those who use a different physician or clinic; or compare the performance and outcomes of a specific physician against the system-wide physician performance profile, and so forth, with all information contoured for the time period selected: a month, a quarter, a year, five years, or longer. Management tools seldom seen before in medical care are now available for use by physicians in "general manager" roles, and by other managers within organized, direct-service systems. In the absence of membership—within a fee-for-service system—it would not be possible to generate performance monitoring and evaluation reports of this kind. The potential for providing the optimal quality of medical-care services within an HMO is already light-years beyond what might be possible under traditional fee-for-service arrangements, where patients basically vote with their feet, and where a firm, longitudinal responsibility by a primary physician for a defined, reasonably stable set of patients is generally impossible to achieve. The fact of membership changes everything. When membership is married with a revolutionary medical information system, and with the primary physician positioned as "general manager," it becomes a practical clinical reality to implement a process of continuous quality improvement within an organized and auditable medical-care delivery system. Simply put, this reality can never be achieved under "Guild Free Choice," fee-for-service arrangements.

Organizing Evaluative Clinical Science

A systematic reconstruction of healthcare information, in combination with the fact of membership, will provide, for the first time in the history of American medicine, the foundation for organizing a thoroughgoing evaluative clinical science. The word "organizing" is used instead of the word "reorganizing" in this instance because this specific dimension of fully rational medical practice—the evaluative sciences—has been virtually nonexistent in contemporary American medicine. The average person, seeing airline pilots going on board with a satchel full of checklists and protocols, and knowing that aviators generally use a checklist and audit method to assure that their performance meets or exceeds established standards, probably would not believe that, by and large, nothing remotely comparable is in use by the medical profession in the United States. The "top guns" of American medicine prefer to fly by the seat of their pants, and they do so most of the time. The means to change this situation lie in the field of evaluative science, applied diligently to clinical medicine. John Wennberg, M.D., said the following in 1992:

> We need a governmental focus on a reform in science policy that brings the evaluative sciences on a par with the biomedical sciences. . . . There is a certain irony that it should be the British National Health Service (NHS) that understands the scope and scale required to establish the evaluative sciences and develop the infrastructure required to learn what works and what patients want. A program is under way in Britain to spend up to 1.5 percent of the NHS budget on outcomes research and the building of networks among providers to manage quality.[26]

Dr. Wennberg was reporting on his testimony before Congress that year in support of increased funding for the Agency for Health Care Policy and Research (AHCPR), arguing that the agency should be given the funds necessary to operate on a broader scale to help "repair the flaws in the scientific and ethical bases of clinical medicine." He observed that "Outcomes research is a classic illustration of how science often begins with the observation of unexplained variation."[27]

It is interesting to note some of the events unfolding during the same period in which Dr. Wennberg testified before Congress about the fundamental importance of evaluative clinical science. The federal agency he was speaking in support of, AHCPR, issued a Health Technology Assessment Report in July 1991 on Carotid Endarterectomy, raising serious questions about the number of these procedures being performed, and about the significant morbidity and mortality resulting from the surgeries, especially those performed on asymptomatic patients. In light of the serious questions raised by AHCPR's panel of experts about the incidence and outcomes of these surgeries, a next logical step in the AHCPR process would have been to issue a formal, detailed *Clinical Practice Guideline,* accompanied by a *Quick Reference Guide for*

Clinicians on the subject of carotid endarterectomy. This surgical procedure had by then become a popular technique for cardiac surgeons in treating patients with transient ischemic attacks (TIAs), asymptomatic carotid stenosis, or stroke. The 1990 Assessment Report estimated the number of these surgeries being performed at 100,000 per year, at an average cost of thirteen thousand dollars per operation. A new "guideline" from AHCPR would have emphasized the findings by panels of medical experts (drawn from academic medical centers and from leading cardiology practices around the nation) that the prevailing use of this procedure reflected wide regional variations, and that:

> there has been no definitive study concluding that asymptomatic patients benefit from carotid endarterectomy. . . . These operations have achieved widespread clinical use even though studies testing the efficacy of the procedure and documenting its associated morbidity and mortality have until now produced conflicting results.[28]

The American Heart Association reported a 1995 estimate of 288.8 carotid endarterectomy procedures per 100,000 citizens in the United States, or over 750,000 such operations in that year. Applying the 1990 cost of $13,000 per procedure, the 1995 outlay for this surgery would approach $10 billion.

More than nine years after the Assessment Report was issued by the agency, a *Clinical Practice Guideline* on carotid endarterectomy has never been published by AHCPR. This may be the result of routine decisions about priorities based on budgetary constraints—AHCPR's annual budget for creating new clinical guidelines is about three million dollars. The other possibility that comes to mind is that, because carotid endarterectomies are prime revenue producers for cardiac surgeons, and despite the serious questions raised by a panel of peers about the quantity, appropriateness, and quality of these procedures being done, lobbyists for the surgeons guild may have gotten a message across to Congress that it would be preferable if AHCPR did not proceed to the guideline stage. There is no evidence to be had that this occurred, only rumors. However, if the rumors happened to be true, that would provide a measure of the status of congressional commitment to an increased use of evaluative science in clinical medicine.

The Horror Story of "Practice-Style" Variation

Writing on the subject of variation in surgical practice, Dr. Wennberg has said:

> Most people view the medical care they receive as a necessity provided by doctors who adhere to scientific norms based on previously tested and proven treatments. When the contents of the medical care "black box" are examined more closely, however, the type of medical service provided is often found to be as strongly influenced by subjective factors related to the attitudes of individual physicians as it is by science. These subjective considerations, which I call collectively the "practice style factor," can play a decisive role in determining what specific services are provided a given patient as well as whether the treatment occurs in the ambulatory or the inpatient setting. As a consequence, this style factor has profound implications for the patient and the payer of care. . . . Physicians in some hospital markets practice medicine in ways that have extremely adverse implications for the cost of care. . . . Whatever the reasons, it certainly is not because of adherence to medical standards based on clinical outcome criteria or even on statistical norms based on average performance.[29]

It should be crystal clear from the foregoing quotation that there is no legitimate scientific basis on which to account for the wide variations in surgical and medical practice that presently determine the scale of healthcare expenditures for the nation. It should be quite clear as well that those surgical and medical decisions currently made by physicians "certainly not because of adherence to medical standards based on clinical outcome criteria," but for some other, nonmedical reasons, can indeed be hazardous to human health. From this vantage point, there would appear to be no reasonable or rational alternative for this society, based upon what is known about contemporary American medicine, than to force a prompt and thoroughgoing reconstruction of medical education and medical practice. Promoting effective and broad-scale clinical evaluative science must be an essential ingredient of this reconstruction. The recipe for change must include universal membership in organized systems such as HMOs. It must also include a revolution in the capture and reporting of clinical information, spearheaded by generalist physicians who are occupying the central position in the new medical cosmos.

Reorganizing Economic Incentives

A reconstructed healthcare system in the United States must also bring about a "reversal of centers" in economic incentives for physicians: economic rewards must be structured to flow from health in the patient, rather than from sickness. Almost a century and a half ago, in 1850, the Sanitary Commission of Massachusetts issued a report that included the following statement:

> One of the most useful reforms which could be introduced into the present constitution of society would be that the advice of the physician should be sought for and paid for while in health, to keep the patient well; and not, as now, while in sickness, to cure the disease, which might in most cases have been avoided or prevented.

Per Capita Payment: Enough Is Enough

Although it has been under continuous and increasingly vitriolic attack by the AMA and the medical guild during this century, prepayment for medical care is obviously an old idea, and one with great wisdom underlying it. As Alexander Leaf, M.D., of the Harvard Medical School faculty has said:

> My philosophy always has been that keeping people healthy is the major reason for having doctors. . . . All the incentives are for the physician to do the high-cost things. . . . Even the most honest of us can't help but be influenced by the fact that an operation will generate a large fee, while prescribing diet and exercise, for example, may produce very little income. . . . If the aim of medicine is to keep people healthy and vigorous and active through a long life, then these (preventive) things are worth doing for their own sake.[30]

Using the AMA's latest announcement on the median income of American physicians as the starting point (i.e., $150,000) per annum, let's look at an illustration of how a capitation system works:

> Assume the following about primary-care physicians who care for HMO members who are under age sixty-five:

- They work 4.5 days per week for 48 weeks per year.

- They see 20 patients per day.

- They average 2.5 visits per member per year.

Result:

- 20 × 4.5 = 90 visits per week

- 90 × 48 = 4,320 visits per year

- 4,325 ÷ 2.5 = 1,728 total members registered

Assume that the annual physician's income is at the AMA's median level:

- Salary = $150,000

- Overhead for HMO= 60% of salary, or $90,000

- Combined = $240,000

- $240,000 ÷ 1,728 total members = $138.88 per member per year

- $138.88 ÷ 12 months = $11.57 per member per month

If the average member over the age of sixty-five requires twice the number of primary-care visits annually as do those under sixty-five, then the monthly capitation paid for these members would be $23.14, and the physician's total membership would be reduced accordingly. For example, if half of the physician's patients were under and half over age sixty-five the doctor would have responsibility for 432 persons over sixty-five, and 864 persons under age sixty-five, for a total patient population of 1,296 rather than 1,728. Physician income would remain constant.

In the event that primary-physician income and overhead required an increase of 20 percent, for whatever reason, the per member per month cost would rise to $13.88. This is an entirely reasonable, rational, and proven approach to the compensation of primary care physicians, and many physicians currently working within these economic arrangements would not willingly accept a change. As the aforementioned pediatrician said: "with capitation the thing is, if it is enough, it's enough."

The big problem in capitation systems has to do with how to compensate the "specialists," and particularly the surgeons. John Wennberg has reported finding huge variations in fee-based reimbursements for Medicare patients in the New England area: "Reimbursement for diagnostic X-ray services differed by 400 percent over service areas, electrocardiogram reimbursements by 600 percent, and total laboratory services by 700 percent."[31]

The capitation methodology works reasonably well with such hospital-based "specialists" as radiologists, pathologists, and even emergency-room physicians, where patterns of use can be reasonably predictable, and the cost of specific services can be reliably estimated. For most other "specialists," the effective alternative to open-ended "cost reimbursement" is a price-based variant called "case rate" payment. For expensive procedures such as bone marrow transplants, cardiac bypass surgery, cataract surgery, and total hip replacement surgery, it has been possible for HMOs to negotiate all-inclusive "case rates" based upon the severity of the specific medical or surgical problem, and on the resources required to manage it. The "case rate" will usually include all physician costs, including anesthesia, and in some instances will include all hospital costs as well. HMOs with large enrollments or "market share" have been able to negotiate "case rates" that represent major savings as compared to the cost of the same services paid for under a "cost reimbursement" approach. The incentive under "case rate" payment, as with the DRG system, is for the supplier to deliver the required care in the most efficient and least costly manner possible. While this approach certainly does not "reverse the centers" in the same sense that per capita payment does, shifting the economic incentive away from profiting on sickness and toward profiting from health, it is nonetheless a major advance over "cost reimbursement." Effective negotiation of capitation agreements for primary care and selected "specialist" services, combined with "case rate" payment for those procedures not covered under capitation arrangements, can form the basis of competitive advantage for an HMO or similar managed-care organization, in terms of the relative cost of care, as well as the relative quality of care. As the new millennium begins, there can be little doubt remaining that approaches to payment for medical care that used to be dismissed as "socialized medicine" now represent valid and valuable alternatives to the traditional fee-based arrangement. Thirty years ago, in November 1967, the National Advisory Commission on Health Manpower concluded its study with no doubt about this truth. The commission included the following statements in its report:

COST OF CARE

A major conclusion of the study group is that the Kaiser Foundation Medical Care Program has been able to achieve significant economies in the use of scarce resources and in the medical expenses of its subscribers. Compared to the California average, Kaiser has significantly fewer hospital beds and physicians per member served; and for roughly comparable medical services, Kaiser expenses per member are 35-45 percent less than the expenses of the average Californian. Not all of this difference represents a true economy of Kaiser. First, Kaiser members obtain some of the medical care outside of the Kaiser Plan, thus reducing Kaiser expense per member. Second, indigents and old persons are under-represented in Kaiser compared to the State's population. Still, after making allowances for these factors, it appears that the cost to the average person who obtains medical care through Kaiser is 20-30 percent less than it would be if he obtained it outside.

QUALITY OF CARE

The quality of care provided by Kaiser is equivalent, if not superior, to that available in most communities. Permanente physicians use standard medical practices and procedures. Patient satisfaction is indicated by the overall flow of patients into Kaiser from competing health plans under the dual choice available to all Kaiser subscribers. The Kaiser Foundation Medical Care Program has achieved real economies, while maintaining high quality of care, through a delicate interplay of managerial and professional interests. This has resulted from structuring economic arrangements so that both professional and managerial partners have a direct economic stake in the successful and efficient operation of the overall program. As a result, there has been created a cost consciousness among the health professionals and a healthcare consciousness among the administrators which enables them to work toward a common goal without either sacrificing or overemphasizing their own points of view.

Lessons for Reshaping Federal Policy

This excerpt from a thirty-year-old report makes clear the fact that it has been known for at least this long that HMOs represent the means to bringing the ratio of active physicians to patients into "normal" proportions, i.e., no more than 150 physicians per 100,000 citizens; and the means to removing the prevailing incentive for the fee-based supplier to increase demand for their services for other than medical reasons.

These two positive outcomes—correcting the present ratio of active physicians to population and "reversing the center" of physician initiative— have already occurred on a significant scale in major metropolitan areas of the United States, and the results in terms of the cost of health benefits for the affected populations are evident. The steps that need to be taken now by the federal government to foster and spread the patterns of change already established in the "high change" areas of the nation are quite clear and distinct: market forces alone will not bring about the required reconstruction; it will be necessary for the Congress and the administration to take action to redirect federal outlays for medical education, for medical research, and for the federal purchase of health-insurance benefits or medical services in ways that will encourage and also enforce timely changes in the current behavior patterns evident in American medicine.

In studying California, Minnesota, Oregon, as well as other parts of the country, reconstructions in the healthcare system have already been accomplished in ways that are directly relevant to the overall need for healthcare reform in the nation as a whole. The failure to act swiftly and resolutely, or to act at all, stems not from a lack of knowledge about what is required in the way of change, but from the fact that the free barons, having recognized the impact of these changes on their medical guild, have invested heavily in preventing any action by the Congress or the federal bureaucrats that would change their current modes of obtaining federal largesse for education, research, or reimbursement for fee-based services provided. From the viewpoint of the American medical guild, demand is to be regulated by the suppliers; there is no money to be made from health and wellness (we must have sickness in order to prosper economically); since no feedback flows from the fee-based system, there can be no accountability, and clinical performance will remain unevaluated; and, finally, unsatisfied patients will continue to simply slink away and go shopping elsewhere. For physician free barons these are the "market forces" that must endure. It is evident that a nationwide system of care based upon group and individual membership would change all of these essentials of fee-for-service medicine, to the profound disadvantage and displeasure of the free barons whose livelihoods depend upon it.

The Reorganization of Competition

Many in government and in the private sector believe that market competition will produce the reforms in medical care that can head off the relentless march toward expenditure levels for health benefits that will eventually bankrupt the nation. If the rate of increase in expenditure during the 1965–1995 period is repeated over the next three decades, the per capita annual outlay for medical care will be $82,000 and the United States will be an economic basket case.

It should be clear from the 2,000 percent increase in expenditure during the last thirty years that market competition on the basis of a fee-for-service system will be a ticket to economic doom. Writing in the *New England Journal of Medicine* in 1978, twenty years ago, Stanford University professor Alain Enthoven provided a stark warning to this effect:

> The tax-supported system of fee for service for doctors, third-party intermediaries, and cost reimbursement for hospitals produces inflation by rewarding cost-increasing behavior and failing to provide incentives for economy. The system is inequitable because the government pays more on behalf of those who choose more costly systems of care, because tax benefits subsidize the health insurance of the well-to-do, while not helping many low-income people, and because employment health insurance does not guarantee continuity of coverage and is regressive in its financing.... Headlines will soon appear proclaiming the latest round of healthcare cost increases. The nation's healthcare spending exceeded $160 billion in 1977.[32]

Sixteen years later, in 1993, with national healthcare spending closing in on $1 trillion annually (a general increase of over 600 percent, and a Medicare increase of over 1,100 percent), Enthoven published a litany of the fundamental flaws in the fee-for-service approach:

> FFS has left us with excess supply in many specialties. Too many surgeons are bad for one's health and pocketbook: they lack proficiency and do too many inappropriate procedures. Organized systems can match the numbers and types of doctors to the needs of their enrolled populations.

> FFS has left us with major excesses in hospital beds, MRI machines, open-heart surgery facilities. At least some systems can match all resources used to the needs of the enrolled population.

(FFS) is characterized by major misallocations of resources. Organized systems can allocate all resources—capital and operating—across the total spectrum of care, including less costly settings.

FFS has led to a costly and dangerous proliferation in facilities for such complex procedures as open-heart surgery (OHS). Such surgery done in low volumes has higher costs and higher death rates than when done in high volumes. In California, OHS is done in 118 hospitals, half of which have annual volumes less than 200. Organized systems concentrate OHS in regional centers with low morbidity rates and low costs.

FFS has failed to create accountability for health outcomes and the outcomes information systems doctors need to evaluate and improve practice patterns. Wennberg and others have shown the very wide variations in the costliness of practice patterns among apparently well-trained doctors. Organized systems can gather data on outcomes, treatments, and resource use, evaluate practice patterns and motivate doctors to choose economical practices that produce good outcomes.

FFS has little or no capability to plan and manage processes of care across the total spectrum (inpatient, outpatient, office, and home). Organized systems do.

FFS "free choice" leaves patients to make remarkably poorly informed choices of doctor. Organized systems select doctors for quality and efficient practice patterns, monitor performance, and take corrective action where needed.[33]

"Managing" the Competition

The foregoing presents the facts about fee-for-service medicine, and about the "Guild Free Choice" principles that have been propelling American society toward a fateful, and potentially fatal, economic reckoning. Annual expenditures of $82,000 per capita may seem unimaginable, yet the forces that produced a 2,000 percent expenditure increase over the past three decades remain largely in place, most particularly in the huge tax-supported programs that are already breaking the federal bank. With the understatement characteristic of a gentleman, Enthoven offers these comments:

Our form of government is very inflexible. It is very difficult and time-consuming to change such things as Medicare law and regulations which have been negotiated with financially and politically powerful interest groups that can block efficiency-improving changes that are to their disadvantage.[34]

What Enthoven views as *inflexibility* may in fact be the exact opposite, i.e., a *flexibility* on the part of federal lawmakers on a scale that would equate with spinelessness, as a response to the various forms and levels of pressure regularly exerted upon them by the "financially and politically powerful" proponents of "Guild Free Choice" and its fee-for-service underpinnings. Nonetheless, because the underlying systemic problems evident in American medicine are not self-correcting, the issue of healthcare reform will remain on the national legislative agenda unless or until concrete, significant progress is made in reconstructing the existing medical cosmos.

If market competition is to play a practical role in reconstruction and reform of America's medical-care system, fee-for-service medicine cannot be a significant ingredient of the marketplace. For all of the reasons that Enthoven has enumerated, the national market competition in medical care must take place between and among several dozen fully competent HMOs or other legitimately organized systems of care.

Enthoven has correctly observed that the key driver of a competitive healthcare system, in which the nature of the competition is itself healthy and fruitful for the society, will be informed consumers who are seeking to obtain "maximum value for money." In proposing "managed competition" as a central feature of the Clinton healthcare reform effort, however, Enthoven argued the need for "agents called sponsors" who would "play a central role in managed competition." More than any other single factor, this idea about "sponsors" gave the opponents of reform the ammunition to bring the Clinton plan down in flames. The national network of HIPCs (health insurance purchasing cooperatives) or CHPAs (consumer health purchasing alliances) seemed to many like the same old alphabet-soup labels for all-knowing, big-government bureaucracies that would solve the intransigent social problems related to medical care, despite clear evidence that the feds' own VA hospitals were poorly operated. Once the plan for a national network of HIPCs and CHPAs was circulated in graphic form, with each of the hundreds of "sponsors" having its own board of directors appointed by the state governor; each having its own executive director with a six-figure salary; each having its own staff of "experts" who would referee "managed competition"; it then became possible for anyone with their ear to the ground to hear hoof-beats galloping toward Washington, bearing the AMA's messenger with a political death warrant for the president's plan. At one point Ira Magaziner, the White House czar of the Clinton healthcare reform plan, issued a typically arrogant dictum that a group purchaser of health-insurance benefits on behalf of between 1 and 5,000 people "would be required by federal law" to buy through one of these "alliances." He added that the "sponsors" would "completely replace the way large insurers distribute their products today." Florida foolishly proceeded to set up eleven of these "alliances" around the state, in the absence of any facts about possible federal action. If the average number of "alliances" had turned out to be just five per state, government would have thereby embarked on a campaign to establish and to "qualify" two hundred and fifty of these "sponsoring agencies" around the nation, in order to distribute health-insurance products to the buying public. All this because of the idea that "sponsors" would be required as an element of reform.

Here is what Enthoven said at the time about the need for "sponsors":

> A sponsor is an agency that contracts with health plans concerning benefits covered, prices, enrollment procedures, and other conditions of participation.

> Managed competition is a purchasing strategy designed to obtain maximum value for money for employers and consumers.

> Managed competition is price competition, but the price it focuses on is the annual premium . . . not the price for individual services.

> To understand managed competition, one must begin with the concept of a sponsor.

> In managed competition, the sponsor has several important functions:

> - First, it establishes and enforces principles of equity.
> - The sponsor must select the participating health plans.
> - The sponsor manages the enrollment process.
> - The sponsor must define the enrollment procedures.

- The sponsor must prepare informative materials about the benefits covered, the characteristics of the health plans and locations of their providers, and summarize relevant information about quality.

- The sponsor establishes contractual payment terms with participating employers and individuals.

- The sponsor runs a clearing house for the money.[35]

With the possible exception of establishing and enforcing principles of equity, it is evident that each of the "several important functions" listed above is already being performed by employers or by health plans themselves. It is nothing less than preposterous to suggest that 250 federally endorsed "alliances" scattered about the nation to take over the performance of these mainly "backroom" tasks would somehow improve that performance, while killing off the existing capabilities in the process. Once the proposed health reforms were put into these terms, the demise of President Clinton's reform effort became inevitable both for the Congress and for the American public.

My own belief is that the concept of "sponsors" or "alliances" has been rooted in a logical fallacy of the most pernicious variety, one that I have dubbed the "fallacy of misplaced simplemindedness." There has been talk for a long time among legislators and healthcare reformers about the need to compel the "consumers" of health services to become "cost conscious." Such talk is usually accompanied by a lot of hand-wringing, and even some self-flagellating, over the role that third-party payment has played in reducing "cost consciousness" on the part of the end users of medical and hospital care. One theory that has many adherents is that if "consumers" are made to pay for their medical care out of their own pockets, the impact of this change would be to force the inflation of prices for health care into line with the inflation in the general economy. This theory gave birth to the idea that the federal government should hand out vouchers to Medicare beneficiaries and Medicaid recipients, to use for the purchase of medical care in the fee-for-service system. A corollary notion about "medical IRAs" has its roots in the same fallacious theory. In American medicine, the fact remains that the suppliers of services—physicians—determine the level of demand for most of those services. Of course, there are exceptions, such as cosmetic surgery. Surgeons actively advertise on television, in magazines and newspapers, in the yellow pages, and even on billboards for cosmetic-surgery patients. This is precisely because it is more difficult to dictate demand in cosmetic surgery. The prospective cosmetic-surgery patient would have his or her suspicions about motive quickly aroused by a surgeon who aggressively suggested nips, tucks, or a nose job, instead of eliciting the concerns and desires of the patient. Surgeons do not advertise for hysterectomy patients, and ads about tonsillectomies are rare. In the case of these two operations, and other "gray area" surgeries, surgeons have not displayed comparable reverence for the preferences of their patient, and the patient is rarely given much choice. In the Wonderland of contemporary American medical economics, these wrongheaded proposals about out-of-pocket payment by "consumers" call forth that fine old British descriptive, balderdash. American "consumers," in general, are not simpleminded.

The fires of rapid escalation in medical expenditures have been raging out of control in this country for over three decades, fueled by the oversupply of "specialist" physicians who have been busily expanding the demand for what they provide; and by a continuous inflow of cash in the form of fees for the services supplied in response to continuously escalating, physician-stimulated demand. The actual increase of 2,000 percent in per capita expenditures that has occurred between 1965 and 1995 cannot be explained by an absence of "cost consciousness" on the part of "consumers." What has taken place has primarily been a radical inflation in *expenditures,* and only incidentally a radical inflation in *prices.* A lack of "cost consciousness" on the part of "consumers" has had little to do with this phenomenon, especially since the "consumer" has had so very little to do with the determination of what is to be supplied in the way of medical care. For these reasons it is imperative to keep clearly in mind the nature and essence of the *competition* that will be required in order to accomplish health reform that can qualify as intelligent. The idea of "sponsors" and "alliances" cannot so qualify.

"Maximum value for money" must be defined in terms of comparative clinical outcomes for the *membership.* Once again, membership changes everything. Population-based information about the *outcomes* of the *management of the processes of care* over an *extended period of time* will be the chief source of comparative advantage for competing HMOs, and will be the principal basis for "consumer" choice among available options. Competition of this nature does not have to be "managed." The health plans providing the health benefits have to be managed exceedingly well, or they will fail to attract or hold members. The maximum value to be gained for premium money will be realized by selecting the plan that displays the best record in terms of maintaining good health among its membership. Within a reconstructed health-care system, maximum value for money will have virtually nothing to do with either price or benefits; it will have everything to do with the documentation of optimal clinical outcomes for the membership as a whole. The nature, essence, and structure of competition must be: who is doing the better job of protecting good health?

In high-change areas where HMO competition has been the most vigorous, differentiation of plans on the basis of price has all but disappeared, as has differentiation on the basis of the configuration of benefits. The HMO market in these parts of the country has evolved to a standard benefit for a standard price, like the airlines. A ticket for first class will cost a lot more, but the differences are not significant enough to keep most folks from using coach. A thoroughgoing reconstruction and reform of the present system of medical and hospital care in America can not be based on increasing "consumer" consciousness about price and benefits. Both will be, and ought to be, pretty much standard, and they will not form a key element of competition. This is why "sponsors" are not needed, and why the competition does not have to be "managed."

What Enthoven has termed a "clearance house for money"—the required "back room" operation for moving premiums to the appropriate HMO for each specific covered family or individual—can be efficiently and economically provided by private-sector third-party administrators or fiscal intermediaries, such as those HCFA uses to handle their massive fee-for-service reimbursement system.

The "spreadsheeting" of competing HMO plans—providing a clear summary of all options available to the group and individual "consumers"— can be provided by the existing network of brokers who serve businesses and private individuals all over the nation. Small businesses and individuals may be required to move to the broker instead of being visited by a broker, so that a "single-door" marketing of all of the qualified health-plan options can be offered in a cost-efficient manner. In addition to displaying comparative benefits and comparative prices for all options, the spreadsheets must display information about comparative performance as measured by the clinical outcomes achieved for each HMO's membership as a whole. Measures of performance must include the quality of administrative service as well as the quality of clinical management of the processes of care. Comparative levels of member satisfaction with the administrative performance of the plan will be a key measure in this regard. Accurate and organized information, regularly included in the spreadsheets describing the competitors, will form the core element of competition within a reconstructed medical and healthcare system.

If competition in a reconstructed system is driven primarily by perceptions of medical quality and administrative services, and by regular reporting of the outcomes for the membership as a whole in terms of each aspect of plan performance, the "consumers" will know precisely what to do, without the aid of a sponsor. If real and verifiable options are provided in terms of population-based comparative clinical outcomes, and in terms of efficient, respectful administrative service, there will be no basis whatever for a fallacious assumption that the average citizen is too simpleminded to identify his or her own best interest; and thereby no basis of need for "managed" competition. The plan with the statistical evidence that it has done the right thing, at the right time, in the right way, using the right resources for all of its members, and which offers standard benefits and price, will win the most members. Build this health plan, and they will come.

On the clinical side of this new outcome reporting, the need will be for accurate, routinely available, membership-based, trended, and severity-adjusted information about all of the results of the processes of care. How well are the patients with chronic disease being managed? How many admissions for "diabetes out of control"? How healthy has the membership been, using measures such as days of work or school missed because of illness? How many members made it through winter without a flu infection? What was the C-section rate? Were any babies lost at birth?

In 1993, after the Clinton health reform plan had been submitted to the Congress, and prior to its political demise, a staff reporter for the *Wall Street Journal* named Ron Winslow wrote a column about the "tumultuous" changes being brought about in health care in Minnesota through the actions of a coalition of major employers. Winslow quoted the vice president for medical affairs of one of the big HMOs in the Twin Cities: "Providers are realizing that in order to compete, they must be accountable. That means joining initiatives that measure how they perform and stack up."[36]

For physician free barons, the measuring of their performance is the beginning of the end for their beloved "Guild Free Choice" approach to doing business. The health benefits officials from Honeywell, Dayton Hudson, Ceredian Corporation, and a dozen other large employers, who were collectively spending over $200 million yearly for their employee health benefits, formed a coalition to pressure competing HMOs to focus on the quality of medical care provided to members, and to provide clear evidence of improvement in clinical performance. Winslow reported as follows:

> The Twin Cities revolution emerged two years ago in the wake of a legislative battle. State lawmakers had proposed a new payroll tax to finance health coverage for Minnesota's 400,000 uninsured residents. Many business leaders were incensed. "It was a plan to finance access to a broken system" says John M. Burns, Honeywell's vice president for health management. . . . During coffee breaks in legislative strategy sessions, a handful of corporate benefits officials swapped tales of frustration over their soaring health costs. Although costs here were nearly 20 percent below the national average, they were rising at 12 percent to 15 percent a year—four times the inflation rate. And these companies had used "every cost-containment trick in the book," says Mr. Hamacher, including negotiated discounts on bills and strict reviews of physicians' decisions. They concluded that more tinkering with the system would be futile and that the approach they were urging on legislators was exactly what they wanted for their employees. Benefits officials formed the coalition in the fall of 1991 and immediately charted their new course. Instead of seeking discounts, they would demand that providers demonstrate a commitment to quality; cost savings, they assumed, would follow. They resolved . . . to purchase care only from an organization that developed and followed its own practice standards and worked to improve overall performance . . . . In an unusual step, the 14 employers agreed to adopt one standard benefits plan to reduce paperwork headaches for doctors. "When purchasers and providers work together to define the product and develop quality standards, that's when you can really start reforming the system."[37]

The fundamental approach taken by this coalition to control the radical inflation of expenditures for medical care was very sound. Because supply is regulating demand in medicine, and because human greed is present in physicians just as it is in other mortals, a startling fact about the $1 trillion-a-year-and-rising American healthcare system is that the more you drive it to quality clinical performance, the more cost-efficient it becomes, as measured by per capita expenditure. There is no other major service system in the culture of which this is true. Quality always implies higher cost, except when it comes to medical care. Organized information provides the key to measuring the quality of clinical performance, starting with primary care information. Improvements in managed-care information systems, and in the reporting capabilities of these new systems, will form the central element of a reconstructed competition among well-managed HMOs, a competition for the loyalty of health care "consumers" over the long term.

The Significance of Clinical Outcome Measurement

To reassure all those citizens who have benefit entitlements through Medicare, FEHBP, CHAMPUS, Medicaid, or other federal programs that HMO membership will be good for them, the national standards required of HMOs to qualify as players in the competition for these members must be reconstructed to include very stringent requirements for the collection and reporting of population-based, severity adjusted measurement of clinical outcomes resulting from management of medical and healthcare processes over time.

There has been a significant fear on the part of HMOs that the plan doing the best job as defined by clinical outcome measures would be punished severely as a result of thereby attracting an adverse risk. For example, an HMO reporting outstanding clinical management of members diagnosed with NIDDM might well attract every diabetic within its service area into joining the plan. It would not be unreasonable to expect a response of this sort, and some provision has to be made to level the field of competition with regard to the average morbidity from one plan to another. J. P. Newhouse, a federal researcher specializing in health-insurance issues, has noted in his paper on "Rate Adjusters for Medicare Under Capitation," in HCFA's 1986 Annual Supplement, that in the study conducted by the RAND Corporation, "the one percent of patients with the highest costs in a given year accounted for an average of 28 percent of total costs." Obviously, there must be a means to adjust for the maldistribution of risk among the competing plans—and in two ways: the payment must be adjusted to provide adequate financing to an HMO that has a membership with higher-than-average morbidity; and, equally important, the population-based statistics must be appropriately adjusted to correct reporting of outcomes for any significant differences in average severity of illness within the membership base of each competing plan, one way or the other.

It is noteworthy that risk-adjustment of this kind, in terms of premium payments or in terms of reports of clinical outcomes, would not be possible in the fee-for-service system of "Guild Free Choice." Membership, and the contractual, longitudinal responsibility and accountability that go with it, are prerequisites of an auditable and justifiable approach to the adjustment of risk. The free barons of American medicine have designed a system in which it would be impossible to do this, and there will surely be a well-financed struggle to protect the current guild system from any reconstruction.

The society has no other legitimate alternative available today than to see this inevitable struggle fully joined, a struggle between its own "highest purposes" and the narrower interests exhibited by the "specialist" physicians of the American medical guild. The society cannot afford to avoid undertaking this struggle, and it also cannot afford to lose. The physicians of America cannot afford to win it; however, in their traditional arrogance most are unlikely to recognize this irreducible fact. In a book entitled *Improving Clinical Practice: Total Quality Management and the Physician*, David Blumenthal, M.D., of the Health Policy Research and Development Department at Massachusetts General Hospital, expresses the insights which must be brought to fruition in a reconstructed medical-care system:

> The happiest and best physicians of the twenty-first century are likely to be those who leave their residencies with the scientific, analytic, and personal skills and attitudes necessary not only to adapt to continuous change, but also to lead continuous improvement in their own practice and settings.[38]

The foregoing is consistent with a new and different scheme of ideas for American medicine, one that requires radical changes in the attitudes and professional behavior of practicing physicians. Establishing this new and different scheme of ideas from the halls of academic medicine to the fields of clinical practice will require nothing less than the reconstruction of medical education, medical research, medical licensure and regulation, and medical practice, thereby vesting power and control in the hands of generalist physicians trained to carry on *the* science of medicine at the point of first contact, and prepared to function effectively as the general managers of America's medical-care system. Society must either aggressively accomplish a reconstruction of this kind or watch as the economic vitality of the unique American experiment is sucked dry by an unreconstructed medical-care system that has already amply demonstrated its potential to bankrupt the nation.

Concluding Precautionary Postscript

Many sincere and meaningful books, intended to bring the need for a radical reform of American medicine to public attention before it kills us, have been shelved and ignored. I have begun with documentation of the fundamentally erroneous conceptual assumptions that American medicine has been built upon, and has clung to, which account for why things have gone so awry. The "worldview" of European feudalism that traveled to Jamestown and Plymouth Rock with the first settlers became as the prevailing cosmology of American physicians during the first two centuries in the New World, a time in which physicians and their apprentices had very limited educational opportunities. Since the first medical school opened its doors in America, the courses traditionally offered have constituted a narrow curriculum, ignoring the traditional "liberal arts" insofar as possible, and concentrating on the *materia medica*. As a direct result, on the threshold of the twenty-first century, the organizational basis of American medicine—the guild—is indebted chiefly to the 350-year-old "worldview" imported to the New World with the early settlers.

I next address the most significant aspects of American medicine that have been, and remain, destructive of the most hallowed Western medical traditions; and then I present an outline for a thoroughgoing reconstruction of the American medical cosmos, intended to correct what has gone wrong.

Caveat Emptor

Admittedly, this writing has been undertaken at a very late stage of the "crisis" in American medicine, and in full recognition of the entrenched power of the American guild to effectively resist and defeat every concerted effort made to bring about true reform of the structures and behaviors of Guild Free Choice. I intend this volume as a warning to society that, without radical reconstruction—from top to bottom, from the selection of medical students to the continuous tracking and reporting of the outcomes of medical interventions—America is going to lose its economic vitality and health.

Unless a reconstruction of truly cosmic proportions is accomplished soon—in medical education, in the arrangement of the medical hierarchy, and in medical practice—the economic foundations of the American experiment will become so badly eroded by the continuing, unrestrained escalation in national expenditures for medical care that financial survival in a competitive global economy will be at risk. Our society cannot weather annual per capita medical care outlays in the range of $82,000. Reaching this outlandish point will require nothing other than a continuation of past and present medical practice. Since not much has changed, and no plans for change are in evidence, annual per capita expenditure on this scale is clearly visible on the horizon. Drastic, radical reconstruction along the lines of the six focal points addressed in this chapter would bring expenditure under control, improve the clinical performance of the physicians, and prevent further erosion of the economic footings upon which American society has been built.

A major social system, medicine, has been designed and constructed by people of limited learning, while relying upon a scheme of ideas that is centuries old, a scheme that, until today, has gone unexamined and unquestioned by America's physicians. The designers of the contemporary medical care system had to cope with a crushing sense of professional insecurity and inadequacy vis-à-vis their German, British, and French counterparts. Early in the century, America's wealthy robber barons, among others, sent their ill family members to Europe, by ship, for appropriate medical care. The defensive response of the free barons of the American medical guild has been to initiate an explosion of "specialism" that has, among other things, all but buried the lofty principles of Hippocrates.

In the world of graduate medical education, the rubric for professors of medicine has been to so intimidate residents preparing for primary practice that, once out in the real world, they will find it difficult to trust their own clinical observations, or to act confidently on the basis of their own direct clinical experience. It would always be safer to refer the problem back to the "center of excellence" in which they were trained. The pedantic myth of the "double blind study" as the only legitimate basis for any action at the primary level not previously detailed in a textbook has had a paralyzing effect on many physicians in family medicine. While the professors in academia doggedly inculcate these insecurities into their students, they are nonetheless fully prepared to establish their own clinical experiments as the "standard of practice" without benefit of any evaluative clinical science at all, much less of a "double blind" study. In the case of surgical procedures, for example, a new departure can be declared to be "standard" after just five or six procedures have been performed. If none of the patients died on the operating table, the surgeon is in a position to declare his new procedure the "standard practice" in that community. Who is to say otherwise? Meanwhile, a physician practicing family medicine who believes that a specific patient would be helped to improved health by taking a daily vitamin and mineral supplement has to consider the fact that peer criticism may result from making this suggestion to a patient in the absence of a "double blind" study that would definitively support such a prescription.

As an aftermath of the 1910 *Flexner Report,* the designers of contemporary American medicine have shoved the generalist physician from the central position in the medical cosmos, and have reclassified generalists as second- or third-class physicians. There has been little or no recognition by the free barons that by pulling off this major political coup they thereby compromised the prospects for *scientific* medicine in America, and redirected the path of medical inquiry firmly in the direction of medical technology. The designers of contemporary American medicine have been more akin to engineers than to architects; more like mechanics than like biologists. The aim and purpose has been to accelerate the pace of technological invention, and the result has been to retard the prospects for scientific discovery and breakthrough. The approach has proven to be a very valuable one in terms of the economic rewards flowing to "specialist" physicians.

The evidence in support of these conclusions is plentiful. By stripping the generalist of status and authority, and by systematically denigrating the clinical significance of primary care, the free barons have virtually eliminated any use of the principal basis of clinical observation on which scientific medicine could possibly be based: the complete record of what occurs with the universe of patients at the point of first contact. The source of scientific knowledge in medicine is clinical observation. The most pervasive, most important field of clinical observation in medicine resides with primary physicians. As McWhinney has stated, "clinical observation . . . is *the* science of medicine." The truth of things in medicine will be determined only "by observing and recording, by classification and analysis." Nonetheless, the designers of contemporary American medicine have consigned clinical observation at the primary level to the category of wasted time, and have judged the insight and awareness gained by primary physicians to be insignificant.

The direct result of these stubborn realities is that *scientific* progress in medicine has been slowed to less than a snail's pace, while technological invention—dressed up by the medical guild to look like scientific discovery—has been exploding. The hypotheses that propel *scientific* discovery arise directly from "general description(s) of observed fact." The major source of factual observation in the field of medicine is in family medicine, or primary care. This major field of clinical observation is the fertile breeding ground for the hypotheses that must emerge as a basis for understanding the wealth of clinical facts observed in the primary setting. As Alfred North Whitehead has observed: "Abstract theory precedes the understanding of fact." In medicine, the hotbed of theory must be clinical observation at the primary level.

Under its prevailing scheme of ideas, however, which dismisses primary care as insignificant and rather bothersome, American medicine has virtually closed off access to the very best source of clinical observation on which fruitful scientific medical inquiry might be based. With this source of clinical insight, awareness, and analysis virtually isolated from academic medicine, there is no practical source of information available for a continuous alteration of medicine's abstractions and classifications on the basis of broad-scale, hard-and-fast clinical observation.

American medicine has thus lost its way as a truly scientific discipline, and is instead fiercely prosecuting a "more-is-better" explosion of technological innovation and invention without the benefit of disciplined clinical evaluation. At the same time, and on this basis, the free baron "specialists" are rapidly propelling the society toward financial ruin through the unrestricted—and unlimited—stimulation of "demand" for their own "high-tech" medical services.

The only source of repair and restoration for medical care in the United States will be a radical reconstruction of the contemporary medical cosmos. Most certainly, this will not be easy to accomplish, and time is clearly running out for America.

Notes

1. World Health Organization, *The World Health Statistics Annual* (1990), pp. 104–108.

2. Ibid., p. 104 (U.S.), p. 108 (U.K.).

3. I. McWhinney, "Family Medicine in Perspective," *New England Journal of Medicine* 293, no. 4 (July 24, 1975): 178.

4. B. Starfield, *Primary Care: Concept, Evaluation and Policy* (New York: Oxford University).

5. M. Carey, "Diabetes Guidelines, Outcomes, and Cost-Effectiveness Study: A Protocol, Prototype, and Paradigm," *Journal of the American Dietetic Association* 95, no. 9 (September 1995): 977.

6. J. Pita, Comments on Lewin-VHI study in the *Journal of Clinical Endocrinology and Metabolism* (April 1994).

7. National Institutes of Health, Report, NIH no. 96–3926 (October 1995).

8. R. J. Rubin, W. Altman, and D. N. Mendelson, "Health Care Expenditures for People with Diabetes Mellitus, 1992," *Diabetes Spectrum* 8, no. 3 (May/June 1995): 147.

9. M. Harris, "NIDDM: Epidemiology and Scope of the Problem," *Diabetes Spectrum* 9, no. 1 (1996): 26.

10. Diabetes Treatment Centers of America, "Diabetes Disease Management: The Cost of Diabetes," DTCA Report (March 28, 1995), p. 2.

11. D. Marrero, "Evaluating the Quality of Care Provided by Primary Care Physicians to People with Non-Insulin Dependent Diabetes Mellitus," *Diabetes Spectrum* 9, no. 1 (1996): 32–33.

12. A. Peters, "Community Diabetes Care: A Ten-Year Perspective," by R. G. Hiss et al., *Diabetes Care* 17 (1994): 1124–34. Commentary by Anne L. Peters, *Diabetes Spectrum* 9, no. 3 (1996): 175.

13. W. Fore, "Diabetes Treatment in a Managed Care Setting," *Diabetes Care* 19, no. 7 (July 1996): 786.

14. World Health Organization, *The World Health Statistics Annual* (1993), p. B-93 (U.S.), p. B-623 (U.K.).

15. Pew Health Professions Commission, "Critical Challenges: Revitalizing the Health Professions for the Twenty-first Century," 3d Report, December 1995, p. xvi.

16. I. McWhinney, "Family Medicine in Perspective," pp. 176–80.

17. Pew Health Professions Commission, "Critical Challenges," p. 10.

18. Ibid., p. 3.

19. Ibid., p. 16.

20. B. Starfield, "Primary Care and Health: A Cross-National Comparison," *Journal of the American Medical Association* 266, no. 16 (1991): 2268–71.

21. Pew Health Professions Commission, " Commission Policy Papers" (April 1994): 2–12.

22. I. McWhinney, "Family Medicine as a Science," *Journal of Family Practice* 7, no. 1 (1978): 55.

23. I. McWhinney, "The Importance of Being Different," 1996 William Pickles Lecture, *British Journal of General Practice* 46 (July 1996): 433–35.

24. A. Enthoven, "Managed Competition in Health Care Financing and Delivery: History, Theory, and Practice," revised paper presented at a workshop sponsored by the Robert Wood Johnson Foundation, Washington, D.C., January 7–8, 1993, p. 2.

25. M. J. Roemer and J. L. Schwartz, "Doctor Slowdown: Effects on the Population of Los Angeles County," *Social Science and Medicine* 13C (December 1979): 214–17.

26. J. Wennberg, "AHCPR and the Strategy for Health Care Reform," *Health Affairs* 11, no. 4 (Winter 1992): 71.

27. Ibid., p. 68.

28. Agency for Health Care Policy and Research, "Carotid Endarterectomy," *Health Technology Assessment Reports* no. 5R (1990), p. 9.

29. J. Wennberg, "Variation in Surgical Practice: A Proposal for Action," in *Surgical Care in the United States: A Policy Perspective*, ed. M. L. Finkel (Baltimore: Johns Hopkins University Press, 1988), pp. 58–59.

30. A. Leaf, quoted in "Is Our Care System Killing Us?" by E. Carlson, *Modern Maturity*, April/May 1984, p. 36.

31. J. Wennberg, "Small Area Variations in Health Care Delivery," *Science* 182, December 14, 1973, p. 3.

32. A. Enthoven, "Consumer-Choice Health Plan," *New England Journal of Medicine* (March 23, 1978): 648.

33. A. Enthoven, "Managed Competition in Health Care Financing and Delivery," pp. 20–22.

34. Ibid., p. 6.

35. Ibid., pp. 8–11.

36. R. Winslow, "Employers' Attack on Health Bills Spurs Change in Minnesota," *Wall Street Journal*, February 26, 1993, p. A1.

37. Ibid., p. 2.

38. D. Blumenthal, *Improving Clinical Practice: Total Quality Management and the Physician* (San Francisco: Jossey-Bass Publishers, 1995), p. 13.

6.

Prolegomenon to Any Future Health-Reform Proposals

The American philosopher and social critic John Dewey once observed that "the most pervasive fallacy of human thinking is the neglect of context." The following compilation of statements and queries is included here in order to flesh out the context within which planners, policy makers, administrators, legislators, educators, and ordinary citizens must reason in order to intelligently develop and evaluate ways of reforming America's health-care system.

Over twenty years ago, in 1976, a federal health official named Dr. Charles M. Croner wrote the following words: "For a nation the function of the health care system is to optimize the prevalence of good health and to minimize the toll of ill health among its citizens."[1] How is it possible for any reasonable person to find themselves in disagreement with any aspect of Croner's statement? How is it possible for a society to "optimize the prevalence of good health and to minimize the toll of ill health among its citizens" when it has placed its faith in a medical-care system that exhibits so many contrary characteristics? Croner's view is consistent with ideas expressed by Abraham Flexner in his 1910 report on medical education:

In modern life the medical profession is an organ differentiated by society for its own highest purposes, not a business to be exploited by individuals according to their own fancy. The physician . . . is a social instrument, and the medical school . . . is a public service corporation.[2]

In response to the publication of the *Flexner Report* in 1910, the medical guild undertook a wholesale reconstruction of medical education and medical practice in the United States. To guide them in the implementation of the reforms proposed by Flexner, America's medical leaders relied upon the dominant and fatally flawed scheme of ideas that they had inherited from Europe centuries before. Alfred North Whitehead described this scheme as follows:

Nature is a dull affair, soundless, scentless, colourless; merely the hurrying of material, endlessly, meaninglessly. However you disguise it, this is the practical outcome of the characteristic scientific philosophy which closed the seventeenth century.[3]

This selfsame and fundamentally erroneous scheme of ideas, which has been further detailed and delineated in earlier chapters, has provided the principal intellectual underpinning of twentieth-century American medicine. From the time that Flexner's report was seized upon by the medical guild as its basis for reforming medical education and practice, a series of critical strategic choices made by America's medical leadership have repeatedly reflected their genesis as being this deeply ingrained and erroneous scheme of ideas. Consistently wrongheaded decisions made in this century by the leaders of the American medical guild have produced the following tangible and highly destructive aberrations:

- There exists a radical oversupply of physicians in the United States. There are at least 225,000 more doctors in practice today than are needed to properly care for the medical needs of the entire population. This oversupply is not diminishing because the overproduction of physicians is continuing, particularly in the "specialties."

- Payment for physician services is predominantly fee-based, within a system in which the suppliers of services are simultaneously the principal regulators of demand for those same services. Physicians define the level of demand for medical, hospital, and ancillary services, and therefore the level of expenditure for medical care.

- In fee-for-service medicine, there is no means by which physicians can benefit financially from health in their patients. Under the predominant fee-based mode of physician compensation in America, it is impossible to realize a profit from the prevention of illness or trauma. For virtually all encounters with a patient, income of any significance for the physician requires the presence of illness or trauma.

- There exists a hierarchical arrangement in American medicine under which surgical "specialists" occupy the highest ranks, and physicians engaged in primary medicine have been consigned to the lowest ranks.

- A perverse bias, flowing directly from this topsy-turvy hierarchical arrangement, has been introduced into the criteria and processes used in selecting medical students; into the content of academic curricula; and into the intellectual climate within which physicians are being prepared to practice medicine, a climate that today defines *primary physician* in pejorative terms.

- Investments in medical research are focused on high technology, a focus which has served to confirm an important observation by A. M. Taylor, who gave the Tallman Lectures at Bowdoin College in 1964–65, and who is professor of physics at the University of Southampton, England. Referring to the contemporary tendency to confuse technology with science, a tendency that has been pronounced in the field of medicine, Taylor warned that: "The handiwork of the craftsman is mistaken for the intellectual creation of the savant."[4]

- There currently exists a careless approach to the collection, management, and reporting of clinical information, which can be seen as endemic to the medical profession.

- Radical and inappropriate variations in "practice style" are being exhibited in the professional behavior of many contemporary physicians.

- Patients are being consistently and persistently denied the opportunity to make an informed choice among treatment options that have been set forth for them in an unbiased manner by the attending physician.

American society has traditionally placed its faith in the medical profession. In view of Flexner's dictum that medicine "is an organ differentiated by society for its own highest purposes," there is a clear right for the society to ask, at the very least, where America's physicians have found their ideas. The following questions present themselves:

How is it possible that modern American medicine could be controlled by a scheme of ideas, and a theory of knowledge drawn from a centuries-old erroneous cosmology? How is it possible that American medicine has persisted in attempting to progress as a science on the basis of so erroneous an epistemology? The human organism, in all its complexity, forms the subject and the object of the field of inquiry known as medicine. The concept of a clockwork, or indeed any mechanical conception, constitutes a perverse and wholly misleading notion to apply to the study of an *organism*. An organism is by nature and essence a *process*, a complex mixture of orderly and unpredictable events moving in directions not always clearly foreseeable, and to incompletenesses not easily predictable. Consider these words of John Dewey:

> We live in a world which is an impressive and irresistible mixture of sufficiencies, tight completenesses, order, recurrences which make possible prediction and control, and singularities, ambiguities, uncertain possibilities, processes going on to consequences as yet indeterminate. They are mixed not mechanically but vitally like the wheat and the tares of the parable. We may recognize them separately but we cannot divide them, for unlike wheat and tares they grow from the same root. Qualities have defects as necessary conditions of their excellencies; the instrumentalities of truth are the causes of error; change gives meaning to permanence and recurrence makes novelty possible. A world that was wholly risky would be a world in which adventure is impossible, and only a living world can include death. Such facts . . . have rarely been frankly recognized as fundamentally significant for the formation of a naturalistic metaphysics.[5]

Such facts have also been rarely recognized as having fundamental significance for a reconstruction of the cosmological notions that drive medical thinking in America today, as well as for a reconstruction in the prevailing medical theory of knowledge. These reconstructions must reshape medical thinking and behavior along the lines of the processive, organic, and coherent scheme of ideas that Dewey has managed to elucidate in six short sentences. An *organic* cosmology and an *organic* theory of knowledge must entirely replace the mechanistic and dualistic scheme of ideas that currently informs American medical theory and practice; and must become the driving force of a new departure for medical inquiry, consciously rededicated to serving "the highest purposes" of this society.

Two themes permeate this book: (a) that the evident crisis in American medical and health care is a crisis of excessive expenditure, caused chiefly by an enormous oversupply of physicians, most of whom are disabled by an erroneous mindset that motivates their professional attitudes and behavior; and (b) that unless these specific current afflictions are accurately diagnosed and effectively treated now, or very soon, the crisis will continue to fester, eventually reaching a point of no return. The experts and public policy wonks have been touting solutions for decades, yet any reasonable evaluation must conclude that the situation has only worsened with time. A radical shift in the prevailing circumstances, in terms of both the oversupply of physicians and the deficiencies in medical mindset, offers the only hope for the salvation of American medicine.

An analogy from the field of biology may prove useful in supporting my contention about the problems that flow from medicine's philosophical underpinnings. It may also help to buttress the finding that the dominant mind-set of today's medical guild is fatally flawed. The Centers for Disease Control's estimate that at least eighty thousand Americans die each and every year from nosocomial infections (i.e., a hospital-acquired infection that is neither present nor incubating prior to the patient being admitted to the hospital) makes these hospital infections the fourth leading cause of death in the nation. In terms of airline travel, it would take a crash *every day of the year* in which 220 people die to reach this same level of carnage. How long would the airline industry last under those circumstances? The CDC goes on to report that, in its estimation, at least half of these deaths could be prevented if the physicians and the staff they supervise would adhere to the established procedures for handwashing in the hospital setting. Forty thousand people each year could live instead of die, and a million others could avoid the ravages of a nosocomial infection if doctors simply washed their hands properly. Since physicians have set up a system in which they have control over all interventions with a hospitalized patient, then whenever and wherever nosocomial infections occur, no matter what the specific mode of transmission may be, the buck must stop with the physicians who staff the hospital in which the infections happen, and they are happening in all hospitals.

Anyone concerned about these disturbing facts of "modern" American medicine ought to ask themselves the following questions: How prepared are today's practicing physicians to understand the challenges being presented in acute-care settings by more and more virulent strains of pathogens, displaying increasing resistance to available antibiotic weaponry? How much awareness do today's practicing physicians have of the issues raised in the field of evolutionary biology about the particular deadliness these bacteria can be capable of when the host they are invading is a patient lying immobilized in a hospital bed?; or about the dangers of nosocomial infections not only killing off tens of thousands of patients each year, but of leading to the spread of particularly deadly pathogens in the outside community, borne and transmitted by "cultural vectors" (i.e., doctors, nurses, orderlies, other employees of the hospital, visitors, discharged patients) from nearly seven thousand acute-care hospitals in which compliance with aseptic procedures has generally been the opposite of strict?

In formulating responses to these questions, which are, after all, life-and-death questions, consider the thought patterns of an outstanding physician, Lewis Thomas, who has classified himself as a "biology watcher." It should be clear from the information about him contained in this book that, in terms of an appreciation of the biological sciences, he is an exceptionally well prepared physician. Footnote 33 containing statements made by Dr. Thomas, at the end of chapter 3, includes the following:

> [T]he genuinely decisive technology of modern medicine, [is] exemplified best by modern methods for immunization against diphtheria, pertussis, and the childhood virus diseases, and the contemporary use of antibiotics and chemotherapy for bacterial infections. The capacity to deal effectively with syphilis and tuberculosis represents a milestone in human endeavor, even though full use of this potential has not yet been made. . . . There are other examples, and everyone will have his favorite candidates for the list,

but the truth is that there are nothing like as many as the public has been led to believe.[6]

Not only is it true that there "are nothing like as many as the public has been led to believe"; the further truth is that, as some epidemic diseases that "modern" medicine has given itself credit for "wiping off the face of the earth." are now roaring back in more virulent forms, it is a rare physician indeed who possesses insight into the ongoing evolutionary processes that alone can explain these highly virulent recurrences of "old" diseases.

I'll use Dr. Thomas, a man who has had an extraordinary education in the biological sciences as well as in the humanities, a man whom David Slavitt has called "full of wonder at the universe, well educated, and admirably cultured," to exemplify the point about rarity. Lewis Thomas has written a remarkable book entitled *The Medusa and the Snail,* subtitled "More Notes of a Biology Watcher." It is a wonder of trenchant insights into the symbiotic phenomena of nature. For example:

> The self-marking of invertebrate animals in the sea, who must have perfected the business long before evolution got around to us, was set up in order to permit creatures of one kind to locate others, not for predation but to set up symbiotic households. . . . The best story I've ever heard about this is the tale told of the nudibranch and medusa living in the Bay of Naples. When first observed, the nudibranch, a common sea slug, was found to have a tiny vestigial parasite, in the form of a jellyfish, permanently affixed to the ventral surface near the mouth. In curiosity to learn how the medusa got there, some marine biologists began searching the local waters for earlier developmental forms, and discovered something amazing. The attached parasite, although apparently so specialized as to have given up living for itself, can still produce offspring, for they are found in abundance at certain seasons of the year. They drift through the upper waters, grow up nicely and astonishingly, and finally become full-grown, handsome, normal jellyfish. Meanwhile, the snail produces snail larvae, and these too begin to grow normally, but not for long. While still extremely small, they become entrapped in the tentacles of the medusa and then engulfed within the umbrella-shaped body. At first glance, you'd believe the medusa are now the predators, paying back for earlier humiliations, and the snails the prey. But no. Soon the snails, undigested and insatiable, begin to eat, browsing away first at the radial canals, then the bor-

ders of the rim, finally the tentacles, until the jellyfish becomes reduced in substance by being eaten while the snail grows correspondingly in size. At the end, the arrangement is back to the first scene, with a full-grown nudibranch basking, and nothing left of the jellyfish except the round, successfully edited parasite, safely affixed to the skin near the mouth.

It is a confusing tale to sort out, and even more confusing to think about. Both creatures are designed for this encounter, marked as selves so that they can find each other in the waters of the Bay of Naples. The collaboration, if you want to call it that, is entirely specific; it is the only species of medusa and only this kind of nudibranch that can come together and live this way. And, more surprising, they cannot live in any other way; they depend for their survival on each other. They are not really selves, they are specific *others*.

The thought of these creatures gives me an odd feeling. They do not remind me of anything, really. I've never heard of such a cycle before. They are bizarre, that's it, unique. And at the same time, like a vaguely remembered dream, they remind me of the whole earth at once. I cannot get my mind to stay still and think it through.[7]

Just a few years after publishing these remarkable insights into a natural world clearly perceived and understood in evolutionary and processive terms, the same man, Lewis Thomas, wrote in his autobiography about his feelings toward his own body after a series of unfortunate, complicated, but happily successful encounters with the medical-care system:

I have seen a lot of my inner self, more than most people, and you'd think I would have gained some new insight, even some sense of illumination, but I am as much in the dark as ever. I do not feel connected to myself in any new way. Indeed, if anything, the distance seems to have increased, and I am personally more a dualism than ever, made up of structure after structure over which I have no say at all. . . . I conclude that the arrangement runs itself, beyond my management, needing repair by experts from time to time, but by and large running well, and I am glad I don't have to worry about the details. If I were really at the controls, in full charge, keeping track of everything, there would be a major train wreck within seconds.[8]

Here we have an example of one of the best thinkers in the field of medicine, a mind funded with a deep understanding of evolutionary biology, a man who, in 1974, wrote that he views the whole earth as being "most like a single cell," and yet his perception of his conscious relationship to the con-catenation of cells which, at any given moment, constitute his own mind/body, is not distinguishable from the erroneous presuppositions of René Descartes, nor from those of the other great seventeenth-century Enlightenment geniuses. When it comes to things medical, Thomas's mind-set turns out to be frankly dualistic and mechanistic. In considering his own body much as a complex clockwork "beyond my management, needing repair by experts from time to time, but by and large running well, and I am glad I don't have to worry about the details," Dr. Thomas seems to have entirely abandoned the driving curiosity which has been a marked character-istic of his study of the rest of nature. The main trouble with such a retreat into dualism and mechanism, given the severe intellectual limitations which these seventeenth-century notions impose on medical thinking here at the dawn of the twenty-first century, is that it will prove impossible to carry on a fruitful course of medical inquiry or to continuously improve clinical prac-tice if the processes of thought and the content of imagination nourishing these thought processes remain rooted in a fatally flawed mind-set, an utterly wrongheaded, nonevolutionary scheme of ideas.

Even among contemporary biological scientists there is a distinct, dis-turbing, and ongoing clash between two competing schemes of ideas, although the frankly mechanistic/dualistic cast of mind is less in evidence. Biologists have recently been writing and speaking in terms of contrasting paradigms when discussing the sources of observed higher virulence in emerging pathogens, whether these are new organisms or "old" organisms. The dispute involving contrasting paradigms in biology inevitably impacts upon decisions in medicine about the optimal approach to the clinical man-agement of the new, complex, and potentially epidemic threats that high-vir-ulence pathogens are now posing to the health of the human community. Consider the historical context spelled out by Paul W. Ewald, professor of biology at Amherst College, and self-described evolutionary biologist:

> For most of the past century, the conventional wisdom in parisitology and epidemiology has been that a well adapted parasite is a benign parasite (parasites being defined broadly to include multicellular, unicellular, and subcellular organisms). This view became firmly entrenched during the

second quarter of this century. Although objections were raised during the middle decades of this century, they had little impact in the face of the more aesthetically appealing paradigm, which advocated evolution toward balanced, stable associations in which parasites succeeded through peaceful coexistence with their hosts. The problem with this conventional view is that natural selection does not necessarily favor peaceful coexistence. Rather, it favors those genetic instructions that are passed on preferentially as a result of the characteristics they encode. If instructions that cause their bearer to exploit host resources more fully are more successfully passed into future generations, then adaptation to the host will be associated with increased exploitation of the host. Insofar as increased exploitation causes increased harm, evolutionary adaptation to the host will result in increased harm to the host. . . . [I]n contrast to the situation during mid-century, this time an alternative theoretical framework grew out of this competing view. Now, at the end of the twentieth century this competing paradigm has replaced the "conventional wisdom" among evolutionary biologists. This fundamental change in our view of host/parasite evolution promises to transform perspectives and research programs in parisitology and the health sciences. This transformation, however, is still in progress, largely because of the viscosity at the interface between disciplines. Even now the tenet that well-adapted parasites are benign is considered by many to be a guiding principle. Parasitologists still often speak of benignness as a sign of a well-adapted parasite or infer that mildness is a sign that a host is a natural host. Similarly, this outdated view has also colored the prevailing interpretations of aspects of infectious diseases, such as the origins and evolution of human immunodeficiency virus (HIV).[9]

For the purposes of this concluding argument, the most important point to be taken from the foregoing paragraph is that a resolution of the differences in view under the two competing paradigms described here by Dr. Ewald will have fundamental relevance to and pivotal importance for the proper clinical management of emerging pathogens, especially in an inpatient environment. Just one year after the publication of his referenced article in the *Journal of Parasitology,* Dr. Ewald summed up the significance of the "alternative paradigm" for effective disease management:

This evolutionary framework . . . explains the diversity of human parasites in a way that contrasts starkly with the traditional view. . . . The modern

view of the evolution of pathogen virulence—specifically its focus on the
tradeoff between costs and benefits to the pathogen from increased host
exploitation—allows control programs to identify and focus on the most
dangerous pathogens (those that can be established with high virulence in
human populations). . . . Disease control could be made more manageable if
the most dangerous pathogens could be singled out for the most intense
study, surveillance, and control efforts. Experts who have addressed this
problem from an epidemiologic but not an evolutionary perspective disagree
about the feasibility of predicting and preventing the emergence of the most
damaging new pathogens. . . . I argue that improved understanding of the
evolution of virulence (defined broadly as the harmfulness of an infection)
can make this goal more feasible in two ways: (1) by facilitating identifica-
tion and blocking of pathogens that represent the greatest threat should
they become established in human populations (e.g., *Yersinia pestis* during
the Middle Ages and human immunodeficiency virus [HIV] during recent
decades) and (2) by providing methods for inhibiting the emergence of particularly virulent variants of pathogens that are already established in
human populations (e.g., the pathogen that caused the 1918 influenza pan-
demic and virulent, antibiotic-resistant *Staphylococcus aureus*). . . . If the most
dangerous pathogens—the future analogs of the causes of AIDS, malaria,
smallpox, tuberculous, and cholera—could be effectively blocked, the effort
against emerging disease would be successful. . . . I propose that integrating
evolutionary principles with epidemiology would enhance our ability to stay
ahead of the curve. Evolutionary insights should increase our ability to distinguish emerging pathogens according to the longterm threat that they
pose and thereby adjust investments in accordance with the threat.[10]

Here we have a biologist with a clear insight into the brute facts about
emerging pathogen virulence, facts that all practicing physicians ought to
have a thorough working knowledge of, informing us in the most genteel of
idioms (such as: "the viscosity at the interface between disciplines"), that a
controversy still persists within his own field about the shift to a paradigm
that the 1859 publication of Darwin's "weird new outlook" ought to have
made inevitable for the biological sciences. It is an unfortunate indicator of
the present state of his field of inquiry that Professor Ewald has taken to
calling the work he has been doing as a scientist "evolutionary biology," evidently recognizing that there are others who view themselves as nonevolutionary, or at least less-evolutionary biologists.

If this is the current state of affairs in the explicitly organismic, processive science of biology; and if a major paradigm shift must yet be accomplished within the field of biology before the "viscosity at the interface" between biology and medicine can be navigated, which is to say before the clinical management of emerging pathogens by physicians can be made more effective, just imagine the relative scale of the analogous challenge of alternative paradigms to be faced in the field of medicine.

Unlike the biologists, however, physicians have given no indication that a serious discussion about alternative paradigms is underway, or is even a matter of concern. It should be possible to conclude from the evidence presented in this volume that the "conventional wisdom" dominating medicine in the United States today has as its intellectual base a scheme of ideas spawned under pre-evolutionary conceptions of nature and of man, conceptions that are at root both mechanistic and dualistic. Replacing this framework of medical perceiving and thinking with an alternative paradigm drawn from the leading edge of conceptualizations formulated since 1859 is going to involve difficult and unpleasant work.

As difficult as it may prove to be to reconstruct the prevailing medical mind-set, starting with the academy and extending to the primary physician's office, omitting nothing in between, there is simply no viable alternative for American medicine if it is to self-correct as any good science should. Recall the eighty thousand deaths each year resulting from nosocomial infections, and listen again to Paul Ewald:

> Emerging hospital-acquired pathogens may pose one of the greatest and most controllable threats to people in countries like the United States, where more than 5 percent of hospital admissions [equating to 2 million patients per year] and about 14 percent of intensive care patients acquire infections during their stay. According to some estimates, nosocomial infections rank among the ten leading causes of death in the United States with dangerous bloodstream infections approximately doubling during the 1980s.[11]

Ewald believes that the threat posed to the outside community by the emergence of hospital-spawned pathogens is far greater than has been recognized, and that these particularly virulent pathogens need to be carefully watched for "their potential to breach by evolution the barriers that have inhibited their broader spread in the past."[12] Will physicians be mindful of the complex yet "most controllable" threats posed by this particularly threatening aspect of the real world of American medicine—the same physicians who have successfully blocked the reporting of the incidence of nosocomial infections? These are the same doctors who have kept the eighty thousand annual deaths caused by these infections out of the federal *Atlas of Morbidity and Mortality* that regularly reports to the public the leading causes of death in the nation. And the same physicians who, as numerous peer-reviewed studies have shown, consistently fail to follow their own established procedures for washing their hands, or for keeping their stethoscopes clean. The same physicians who believe firmly that they provide the best medical care in the world. My answer is, not without a radical and thoroughgoing reconstruction of the dominant physician mind-set, shifting from a mechanistic and dualistic scheme of things to a clearly organismic and processive framework for thought and action.

Notes

1. C. Croner (ed.), "The Nation's Use of Health Resources," DHEW Publication no. HRA 77–1240 (1976), p. 1.

2. A. Flexner, *Medical Education in the United States* (Boston: Updike & Co., 1910), p. 6.

3. A. N. Whitehead, *Science and the Modern World* (New York: Free Press, 1957), p. 54.

4. A. M. Taylor, *Imagination and the Growth of Science* (New York: Schocken Books, 1970), p. 1.

5. J. Dewey, *Experience and Nature* (New York: Dover Books, 1958), pp. 47–48.

6. L. Thomas, *The Lives of a Cell* (New York: Bantam Books, 1975), pp. 35–42.

7. L. Thomas, *The Medusa and the Snail* (New York: Bantam Books, 1979), pp. 3–5.

8. L. Thomas, *The Youngest Science: Notes of a Medicine Watcher* (New York: Viking Press, 1983), p. 232.

9. P. W. Ewald, "The Evolution of Virulence: A Unifying Link between Parasitology and Ecology," *Journal of Parasitology* 81, no. 5 (1995): 659–69.

10. P. W. Ewald, "Guarding Against the Most Dangerous Emerging Pathogens:

Insights from Evolutionary Biology," *Emerging Infectious Diseases* 2, no. 4 (October–December 1996): 245–54.

11. Ibid., p. 252.
12. Ibid., p. 253.

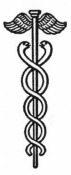

Index

Adjusted Average Per Capita Cost (AAPCC), 189–90, 192, 194–96
Agency for Health Care Policy and Research (AHCPR), 237–38
Almagest, 28–29
American Medicine and the Public Interest, 151
AMNews, 10, 12, 18, 139
amoxicillin, 90
Anderson, R. M., 209
anesthesia, 97
Aquinas, Thomas, 49
Aristotle, 25, 26–28, 30, 49
Armey, Dick, 9, 166
asepsis, resistance to, 77–85
Atlas of Morbidity and Mortality, 275
Atlas of United States Mortality, 85

Bacon, Francis, 41, 62, 63
bacteriology, 81
Barnard, Christian, 108, 128
Blaser, Martin, 89
Blumenthal, David, 255

Boorstin, Daniel, 29, 30, 32, 33, 35,
    36, 42, 43–44, 50, 68, 69
Borelli, Giovanni, 43, 69
Brahe, Tycho, 25, 35, 36
British National Health Service
    (NHS), 237
Broad, C. D., 41
Burtkowski, Peter von, 74
Burtt, E. A., 69
Bush, George, 184
Butterfield, Herbert, 69

California Public Employees Retire-
    ment   System   (CALPERS),
    185–89
Caper, Philip, 235
capitation payment arrangements,
    11, 140, 240–43
cardiovascular disease, 108. *See also*
    coronary artery bypass surgery
Carlson, Rick J., 70
carotid endarterectomy, 128, 238
Center for Policy Studies, 183–84
Centers for Disease Control and Pre-
    vention (CDC), 84, 87, 267
    Hospital Infections Program, 87
Century of the Surgeons, 79
Chassin, M. R., 159
Cherasky, Martin, 13–14
Chrysler Corporation, 216–17
clinical outcome measurement, 254
Clinton healthcare reform effort, 247
clockwork universe. *See* cosmology,
    mechanistic
competition in healthcare, 251–52
Comprehensive Health Planning

(CHP) legislation, 180–81
Copernicus, 25, 33–35, 39, 47, 60,
    62, 67, 91
coronary angioplasty (PTCA), 128
coronary artery bypass surgery
    (CABG), 127–28
cosmology, 15, 24–55, 58, 59–63,
    173, 264
    current medical, defective, 125
    geocentric, 26–32, 59–60
    heliocentric, 33–40
    mechanistic, 40–43, 68–77, 91,
        94
    organic, 46–49, 94
cost of medical care. *See* medical care,
    cost
Council on Medical Education of the
    American Medical Association,
    76
*Critical Challenges: Revitalizing the
    Health Profession for the Twenty-
    First Century,* 217–18
Croner, Charles M., 263

Dale, Henry, 34, 42
Dante, 25, 29–30, 62, 71
*Dartmouth Atlas of Health Care in the
    United States,* 159, 162
Darwin, Charles, 25, 46, 47, 72, 74,
    75, 162, 273
Darwin's Dangerous Idea, 49
Davis, W. K., 209
death
    definition, 103, 107
    major causes of, 85, 211
Debakey Commission, 178

Dennett, Daniel, 46–47, 49
Department of Health and Human Services (HHS), 85
Descartes, René, 25, 37, 40, 42, 45, 62, 67, 68, 69, 71, 75, 76, 91, 104
Dewey, John, 263, 266, 267
diabetes mellitus, 125–26, 173, 205–13, 235–36
diagnosis related group (DRG), 161–62, 182–84
diphtheria, 129
Discoverers, The, 68
diseases, incurable, 94, 129
Dobzhansky, Theodosius, 48
Drucker, Peter, 123, 224

education, medical, 169–70, 257–58
  apprenticeship, 63–65, 66, 71
  proprietary medical schools, 65–66
  reconstruction, proposals for, 94–102, 119–22, 202, 220–23
  university-based medical schools, 71, 80, 162–65
Edwards, A. B., 170–71
Einstein, Albert, 25, 50
End of Medicine, The, 70
Enthoven, Alain, 64–65, 245–49
epistemology, 25, 173
evolution, 48
Ewald, Paul, 129, 271–74

Fabius, Raymond, 211
fallacy of misplaced concreteness, 171–73, 210
Faraday, Michael, 50–51
Federal Employees Health Benefits Program (FEHBP), 186
fee-based medicine, 143
Flexner, Abraham, 66, 76, 94–95, 129, 214, 220
Flexner Report, 22, 74, 95, 97–102, 180, 204, 258, 264
Florida health system, 248
Ford, Gerald, 180
Freud, Sigmund, 72
Furse, Elizabeth, 207

Galileo Galilei, 25, 37–40, 62, 67, 71, 79, 91
Gallup polls, 47
general practitioners, 96
Gentleman, Jane, 127
Geulinex, Arnold, 68
Ginzberg, Eli, 165
gloves, surgical, 80–83, 87–88
Graduate Medical Education National Advisory Committee (GMENAC), 165, 167
Griffin, Katherine, 84, 88
guidelines, practice. *See* practice guidelines

Hall, John, 105
Halsted, William Stewart, 80–82
Harris, Maureen, 208
Harvard Medical School, 80
Harvey, William, 25, 40–42, 72
Head to Head, 14
Health Care Financing Administra-

tion (HCFA), 18, 188, 193

Health Care in Transition, 149

health maintenance organizations (HMOs), 21, 141, 229–36, 251–52

enrollment, 10, 229

Health Professions Educational Assistance Act, 178

Health Systems Agencies (HSAs), 181–82

heliobacter pylori, 15, 89, 126, 176

heredity, 48

Hess, G. E., 209

Hill-Burton Act. *See* Hospital Survey and Construction Act

Hill-Harris Act. *See* Hospital Survey and Construction Act

Hillman, Alan, 12

Hippocrates, 12–13, 26–27, 106

Hippocratic oath, 13, 63, 65

Hiss, R. G., 209

Holmes, Oliver Wendell, 78, 81, 83

Hooke, Robert, 44, 45

hospital capacity, 151, 154

Hospital Survey and Construction Act, 148, 149, 150–51, 152, 154, 157

How to Avoid Unnecessary Surgery, 153

Hubble, Edwin P., 51–52

human immunodeficiency virus (HIV/AIDS), 85

hysterectomy, 112, 115

iatrogenic illness, 82–88. *See also* nosocomial infection

iatrophysics, 69

Improving Clinical Practice, 255

income, physician, 10, 18, 112, 240–43

infant mortality rates, 152–53, 164

Jarvis, William, 84

Jenner, Edward, 73

Johns Hopkins Medical School, 80–81

journalism, 110–12

Kaiser Health Plan, 10, 21, 61, 185, 243

Kepler, Johannes, 25, 36–37, 38, 45, 68

Leaf, Alexander, 240

life expectancy, 199–200, 214

Lister, Joseph, 81, 83

Listerism, 80

Lives of a Cell, 53, 133–37n. 33

lobbying (AMA), 144

lupus, 145

McBurney, Charles, 82–83

McClure, Walter, 183–84

McKeown, Thomas, 70

McWhinney, Ian R., 172–77, 204, 214–15, 220–22, 259

Magaziner, Ira, 248

malaria, 129

Malpighi, Marcello, 25, 43–44

managed-care plans. *See* health maintenance organizations

market forces, 11

Marrero, David, 208

Marshall, Barry, 15, 88–90, 126, 176
Masterson, James F., 88
Mathematical Principles of Natural Philosophy, 42
Maxwell, James Clerk, 51
Medical Assistance Reform Act of 1979, 166
medical care
  access to, 102, 159
  cost, 16, 17–21, 167–68, 178, 187–97, 207, 245–54
  improvements in, 124, 213–14
  inadequate, 125–31, 152–53, 215, 227–29
  payment, mode of, 17, 161–62, 240–43, 249
  per capita cost, 14–15, 19–20, 146–47, 187, 201
  primary-care physicians, 203
  purpose, 102
  reconstruction of, 21–23, 201–202, 221–32, 245–60, 263–75
  supply and demand, 16
Medical Economic Index (MEI), 193
Medical Family Tree, 74, 75
medical records, 223–25, 228–29, 236–38
medical schools. *See* education, medical
Medicare, 20, 155–58, 183–85, 187–88, 245. *See also* diagnostic related groups
Medusa and the Snail, The, 269
Metaphysical Foundations of Modern Physical Science, 69
metronidazole, 90

microscope, 46
Millman, Marcia, 107
Mills, Wilbur, 156
Morrow, J. H., 170–71
Muller, H. J., 48

Nader, Ralph, 179
National Center for Health Statistics (NCHS), 85, 86, 151
National Health Planning and Resource Development Act, 181
National Institutes for Health (NIH), 207
National Nosocomial Infection Surveillance System (NNIS), 85, 86
New England Journal of Medicine, 171, 245
Newhouse, J. P., 254
Newton, Isaac, 42, 44, 62, 67, 68, 69
New Yorker, The, 88
Nixon, Richard, 179–80
North, John, 29, 31, 42, 50, 51, 52–53
nosocomial infection, 82–88

On the Limitations of Modern Medicine, 70
Oresme, Nicole d', 31, 68
organ transplants, 92, 107
Origin of Species, 72, 74, 162
oversupply of physicians. *See* physicians, surplus

Pantin, C. F. A., 46
Paracelsus, 32–33, 63

Pasteur, Louis, 25, 46, 72, 83
pathogen virulence, 130
patient records. *See* medical records
per capita cost of medical care, 14–15
Permanente Medical Group, 10
Peters, Anne L., 209
Pew Health Professions Commission, 17, 19, 168, 194, 213–19
physicians
   ratio to population, 100, 243–44
   surplus, 16, 17–19, 21, 72, 102, 139, 168, 264
Pita, Julio, 206
Polanyi, Michael, 54, 175
poliomyelitis, 92–93
Pope, Alexander, 42
Popper, Karl, 58–59
practice guidelines, 116
practice style, 112–18, 127–28, 153–54, 160, 164, 239
Primary Care: Concept, Evaluation, and Policy, 205
Professional Standards Review Organization, 179
Prospective Payment System (PPS), 182
prostatectomy, 112, 115
protocols for cleanliness (hospital), 130
Ptolemy, 25, 29, 30, 34, 35, 59, 62, 67, 91

radiation therapy, 117
radiology, 11, 227
Randers-Pherson, Justine Davis, 81

Reclaiming Our Health, 78–79
reconstruction
   of medical care. *See* medical care, reconstruction
   of medical education. *See* education, medical, reconstruction
reversal of centers, 217, 220, 224, 227, 244
Richmond, Julius, 73
Robbins, John, 77–79
Roemer, Milton, 152
Roos, Leslie L., 118
Roosevelt, Franklin D., 155–56

Sabin, Albert, 93
scheme of ideas. *See* cosmology
Scientific Developments of the Early Nineteenth Century, 72
Semmelweis, Ignaz, 79–83
Shinto belief, 107
Simon, William, 180
Slavitt, David, 269
Social Transformation of American Medicine, 155, 179
Somers, Anne R., 149–50
specialization, medical, 74–75, 95–98, 168
Starfield, Barbara, 205
Starr, Paul, 155, 158, 179, 181
Stepien, C. J., 209
Stevens, Rosemary, 151
stomach ulcers, 15, 89, 126
stroke, 238
Study of Surgical Services in the United States (SOSSUS), 170, 171

Surgeon's Glove, The, 81–82
surgery, discretionary, 127, 249
surgery, unnecessary. *See* practice style
Surgical Care in the United States, 118–19

Tax Equity and Fiscal Responsibility Act (TEFRA), 189, 192–93
Taylor, A. M., 53
Taylor, F. Sherwood, 72
technical proficiency, 117–18
technology, medical, 91, 92–94, 133–37n. 33, 228–29
Thomas, Lewis, 53, 92, 93–94, 268–71
Thorwald, Jurgen, 79, 81
Thurow, Lester, 14
tonsillectomy, 112, 114
training of physicians. *See* education, medical
Truman, Harry, 156
tuberculosis, 129

ulcers. *See* stomach ulcers
universal healthcare bills, 156
Unkindest Cut, The, 107

Vesalius, 40, 62

Wagner, Robert, 155
Warren, J. Robin, 88
Washington Post, 20
Wennberg, John, 107, 112, 114, 159, 160–61, 235, 237, 239, 242
Whitehead, Alfred North, 39, 54, 58, 59, 76–77, 171, 259, 264
Williams, D. C., 171
Williams, Lawrence, 153
Winau, Rolf, 74
Winslow, Ron, 252
World Health Statistics Annual, 199–200

Zantac, 90